Sex and Sexuality in Ancient Greece

Sex and Sexuality in Ancient Greece

L J Trafford

PEN & SWORD
HISTORY

First published in Great Britain in 2026 by
Pen & Sword History
An imprint of Pen & Sword Books Limited
Yorkshire – Philadelphia

ISBN 978 1 39903 225 4

A CIP catalogue record for this book is available from the British Library.

Typeset by Mac Style
Printed in the UK by CPI Group (UK) Ltd, Croydon, CR0 4YY.

FSC
www.fsc.org
MIX
Paper | Supporting responsible forestry
FSC® C013604

The Publisher's authorised representative in the EU for product safety is Authorised Rep Compliance Ltd., Ground Floor, 71 Lower Baggot Street, Dublin D02 P593, Ireland.
www.arccompliance.com

For a complete list of Pen & Sword titles please contact:

PEN & SWORD BOOKS LIMITED
47 Church Street, Barnsley, South Yorkshire, S70 2AS, England
E-mail: enquiries@pen-and-sword.co.uk
Website: www.pen-and-sword.co.uk
or
PEN AND SWORD BOOKS
1950 Lawrence Road, Havertown, PA 19083, USA
E-mail: uspen-and-sword@casematepublishers.com
Website: www.penandswordbooks.com

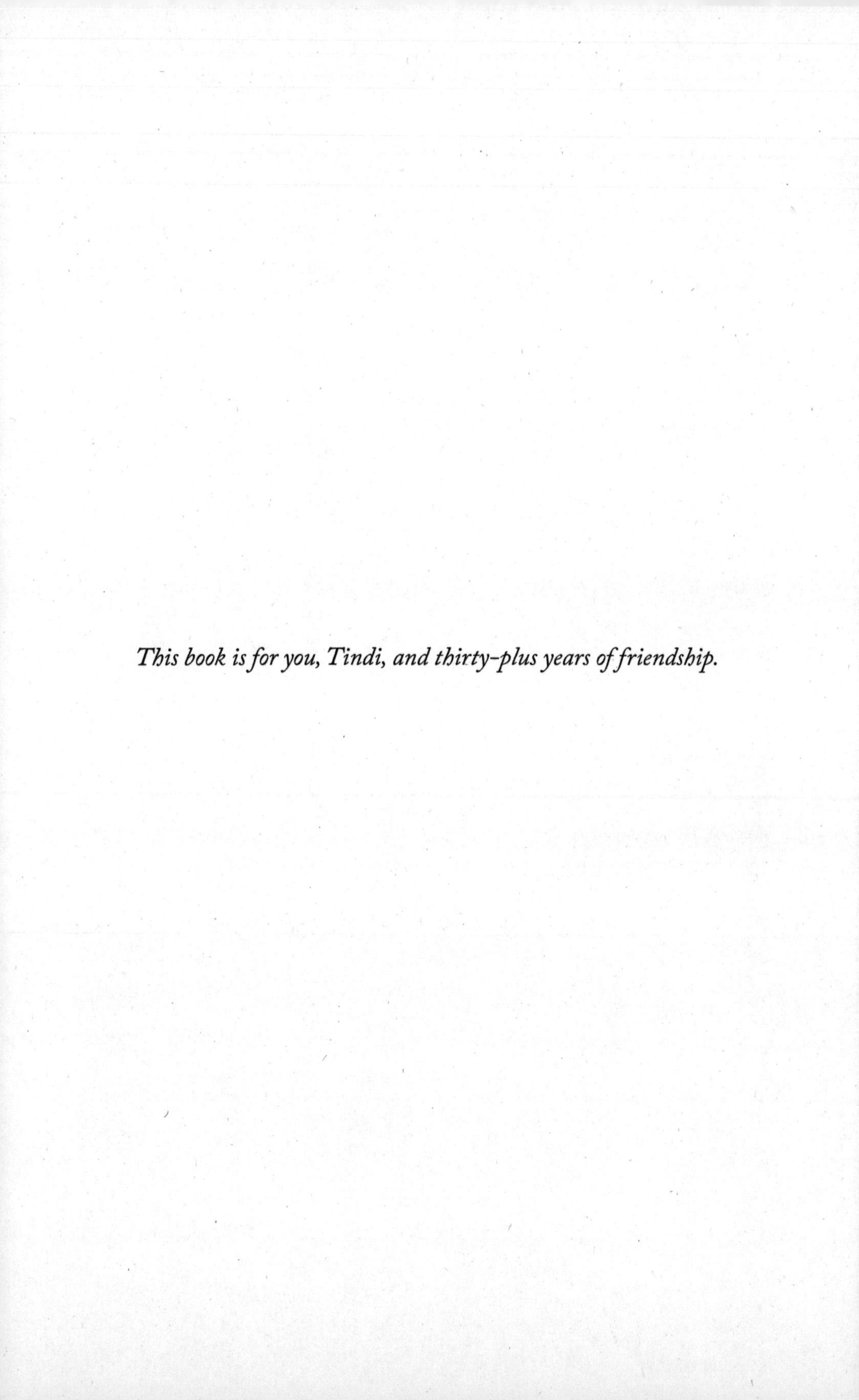

This book is for you, Tindi, and thirty-plus years of friendship.

Contents

Part I

Understanding Ancient Greece

Introduction

Greeks Bearing Gifts

It is the ancient Romans that have the reputation for sexual depravity with their debauched emperors and their round-the-clock, or rather round-the-sundial orgies. It's not an entirely undeserved reputation given the types of artefacts they left behind: filthy frescoes, graphic graffiti and hundreds of depictions of penises to be found everywhere Rome touched. From the heat of the Syrian desert to the cold, damp mist of Hadrian's Wall, Rome was a society that shoved sex in your face. But this is not a book about sex and sexuality in ancient Rome, because I've already written that book.[1] This is a book about sex and sexuality in ancient Greece.

Sex doesn't instantly spring to mind when you think about ancient Greece. Instead, you're likely picturing a group of men with fabulously bushy beards discussing weighty topics like politics, philosophy, art, medicine and what it means to be human. You've probably heard ancient Greece referred to as the 'cradle of western civilisation', the place where much of what underpins our own society was first created. You're likely thinking ancient Greece was a very serious place and the ancient Greek people were very clever. You're not wrong on any of this.

It is from ancient Greece that we get the Hippocratic[2] Corpus, a collection of observations on the symptoms and treatment of the sick, and what the outcomes were for the patient after treatment. The Hippocratic Corpus, as well as being a guide to the human body, its various working parts, the diseases it might face and advice on how to keep those parts healthy, is also where get the key principles of modern medicine. The Hippocratic Oath, first adhered to by doctors living over 2,000 years ago, underpins modern medical practices. Qualifying doctors still swear to uphold this oath, its most famous clause being: do no harm.

It's also in ancient Greece that we find the first democracy, Athens, a society whose values are reflected in the United States of America's constitution: a government of the people, by the people, for the people.

But it's not just words and concepts we have nicked from those clever ancient Greeks, we nicked their stuff too. Go round any major museum in Europe and beyond and you will find at least one room stacked full of sculptures, friezes, busts and vases from ancient Greece, much of which modern-day Greece would really like to get back.[3]

'We are all Greeks. Our laws, our literature, our religion [sic], our art have their roots in Greece. But for Greece … we might still have been savages and idolators.'[4] So said the nineteenth-century Romantic poet, Percy Bysshe Shelley. Shelley was far from alone in his love of the ancient Greeks, his friend Lord Byron was similarly entranced by the achievements of ancient Greece. 'Ancient of days! august Athena! where, where are thy men of might? thy grand in soul? Gone – glimmering through the dream of things that were; First in the race that led to glory's goal, They won, and pass'd away – Is this the whole?'[5]

If you think that's gushing praise, prepare yourself for the introduction to a work that influenced Romantics like Shelley and Byron, *The Art and Architecture of Ancient Greece* by James Stewart and Nicholas Revetts: 'They distinguished themselves by a pre-eminence and universality of genius unknown to other ages and nations.'[6] Geniuses, the whole damn lot of them.

Reverence is the order of the day; we revere the ancient Greeks. You can tell this by how much of their culture we have taken for our own, such as theatre and athletics. We talk just as their earliest philosophers did about what it is to be stoic and we have stolen their ideas on how countries ought to be governed, trumpeting and exporting that across our world as an ideal. We have even taken their words, an estimated 150,000 of them, into our own language, English, and a phrase too: beware of Greeks bearing gifts.

That phrase originates from the time of the Trojan War, a ten-year-long conflict between Greece and the city of Troy (which was situated in what is now Turkey) sometime in the twelfth or perhaps eleventh century BCE or perhaps not in any century, because the story of Troy comes straight out of Greek mythology. To break the deadlock of this (perhaps real) seemingly never-ending war, the Greeks constructed a wooden horse which they parked outside Troy's city walls with a big note tied round its neck saying something along the lines of: 'You Trojans are ace fighters. Better than us Greeks for sure. So we give up. Bye, lots of love the Greeks. P.S. We made you this fabulous wooden horse to say sorry for the past decade we've spent killing and maiming your civilians.'

The Trojans weren't entirely stupid, they sent men down to the shoreline, where the Greek army had been camping out, to check that they had really given up and gone home. They found the camp deserted, there was not a Greek to be seen. They really had gone. Jubilation followed and a big party was held, at which the guest of honour was the huge horse the departing and defeated Greeks had gifted them.

You'll know the twist in this tale. The Greek camp was indeed entirely devoid of Greeks, but not because they had all given up and sailed home. The Greeks were at that very moment sitting inside the belly of that giant wooden horse that the Trojans had naively wheeled into their city. After ten long years, they had finally penetrated Troy's walls without the need for a single siege engine or barrage of spears.

When darkness fell, the Greek army crept out of their hiding place and beat the crap out of the Trojans. Not content with killing the people of Troy, the Greeks wreaked destruction on the city itself. When they had finished their devastation there was little left standing of Troy; it may as well have never existed.[7]

We are a bit like those Trojans, for we too have received a gift from the Greeks, although it's not a wooden horse this time but instead the gifts of art, literature, medicine, science, philosophy that have all influenced our world for the better. So brilliant are the ideas that come from ancient Greece, so enthralling, so captivating that we don't see certain other aspects of ancient Greek society. These are the parts of ancient Greece we didn't willingly absorb into our own culture or gush over in verse. They are the hairy-arsed soldiers crouching in the darkness of the wooden belly of that horse, if you will.

Take Greek theatre as an example, words that conjure up images of the great tragedies such as *Medea* or *Oedipus Rex*, two works that cover grand themes of hubris, revenge and man's helplessness to thwart the pernicious power of the gods. Now let me quote you a few lines from a play written by an award-winning playwright at the height of his highly successful career during this same age of geniuses that created *Medea* and *Oedipus Rex*.

Mnesilochus: Still having difficulties with the dress. Come on, mate, help me. It won't go over my legs.

Thrata helps him tuck his phallus under the dress. The girdle fastens the phallus to his stomach.

Euripides examines the result.[8]

The play is called *Thesmophoriazusae* or, in English, *Women Celebrating the Festival*, and it is worth taking a moment now to appreciate and marvel at this stage direction here. It certainly knocks Shakespeare's *exit pursued by bear*[9] so far out of the ballpark it's interrupted a synchronised swimming event in another country.

That these actions are spelled out in the direction tells you just how keen the director of this particular production of the *Thesmophoriazusae* was to milk every knob gag he was served up in the text by its author. There are a lot of knob gags in *Thesmophoriazusae*, aided by the plot which involves the male Mnesilochus disguising himself as a woman to infiltrate a woman-only festival. That all the female characters would also be played by men adds to the humour of Mnesilochus' attempts to blend in. Also aiding the joke were the costumes the actors would be wearing, which included fake oversized phalluses. You can imagine the laughs a good actor could get out of a floppy costume penis.

Ancient Greece is a surprising place, a place as duplicitous as that beautifully crafted wooden horse. It's a duplicity we created in gazing only upon the gifts and ignoring everything else that came with those gifts. Sex and sexuality is definitely a hairy-arsed Greek soldier of a topic, so you'd better prepare yourselves to be surprised as we take a tour around an alien world where ordinary everyday activities are done completely starkers, penis cakes are baked for a key public holiday and where we shall stumble across some of the most explicit and pornographic images you're ever likely to see (even in an internet world!) depicted on the ancient equivalent of a coffee mug. Kick those bearded philosophers and those oh-so-clever men firmly on the ankles because it's time to get acquainted with the real ancient Greeks.

Chapter 1
The Basics

I very unsubtly hinted in the introduction to this book that the ancient Greece we're going to be examining is going to be very different to the ancient Greece you think you know. Our image of ancient Greece is rather like a chocolate box where the second layer has been raided for strawberry creams and smooth pralines whilst there's still coconut eclairs on the first layer. There are a lot of coconut eclairs in ancient Greece, and it's time to pop them in our gobs and do a hard swallow. I'll be on hand with a glass of water, for there are going to be some very hard swallows in this book, because the ancient Greece we think we know, it turns out, we really don't.

But before we get to chew on those coconut eclairs, we need to ask what will seem like some very obvious questions to you, but stay with me because like everything connected to ancient Greece they are more complex than they first appear.

What is Greece?

Today everyone knows that Greece is the knobbly bit to the right of Italy along with all those specks of islands in the Mediterranean Sea that make a very pleasant holiday destination for millions of us each year. But that knobbly bit and accompanying specks (all 227 of them) only came to be one country in 1830. Before then it had enjoyed an interesting history that had seen it become part of and then break away from country-swallowing empires such as the Romans, the Venetians and the Ottomans. Predating all of these in the fourth century BCE, a certain dashing young adventurer named Alexander came down from Northern Greece and began his own country-swallowing empire, earning himself an extension to his name, 'the Great'. Humble he was not.

For most of its history, Greece was not a singular country at all, nor did it think of itself as one. The ancient Greece we will be looking at was made up of hundreds of city states, some of which were not even located in what we think of as Greece today. The Greeks were early colonisers and colonies of people who thought of themselves as Greek were to be found across the Mediterranean basin in Italy, Sicily, Turkey and North Africa.

Some of these city states we shall be looking at you will have heard of before, states such as Athens and Sparta which loom large in history. Other city states from this era you'll have heard of accidentally, because they've given their names to UK-wide shopping brands such as Argos, spotty dogs such as Dalmatia, and a sexual orientation such as the island of Lesbos. The remaining many hundreds will likely have passed you by. Ever heard of Euboia or Megara? Didn't think so.

These city states were diverse in their political structures, their societal set ups, their attitudes towards sex and sexuality and what evidence they left behind helpfully describing any of this. Possibly this is because they spent most of their time fighting each other for supremacy and nobody had the time to document these matters, being otherwise engaged in killing each other. However, it was a fight with an outsider that brought these diverse squabbling city states together and it is from this battle that we first see the emergence of a shared identity, that of being Greek.

In 480 BCE, these small battling city states faced a larger threat than any of them had ever encountered before; the mighty Persian Empire and its King of Kings, Xerxes. The ancient Greek historian Herodotus, who was a very near contemporary to these events, having been born around 484 BCE, lays it on thick as to how mighty the Persian forces that invaded Greece were. Herodotus claims that the Persians had an army of 2.5 million men. Modern historians are far more cautious and vaguer with their estimates; they believe the Persian forces to be in range of 200,000–500,000 men due to complicated calculations involving the logistics of recruiting, moving and feeding an army. Though, even if we accept their lowest estimates of an army of 200,000 men, this is still many times the size of the combined Greek forces they faced.

During this war, the Spartans were sent word from the Persian king who was busy fighting the Athenian navy far away from the Spartan homeland.

Athens was certainly no ally of Sparta, but in a fight between Persia and Athens the Spartans looked at the eastern invaders and they looked at the Athenians defending their land and something new arose in their hardened man chests. It was a feeling of solidarity with Athens, a feeling that they had more in common with them than the Persians. A feeling we might call 'Greekness'.

The Spartans explained this new feeling of theirs to the Persian ambassador.

> The kinship of all Greeks in blood and speech, and the shrines of gods and the sacrifices that we have in common, and the likeness of our way of life, to all. Know this now, if you knew it not before, that as long as one Athenian is left alive we will make no agreement with Xerxes.[1]

Which is all very stirring and moving and in the film version will be accompanied by a soaring soundtrack and cheers from the audience. Best to ignore the epilogue where this newfangled idea of being Greek was easily shed as the forces of Sparta and Athens, who only a few decades before had stood together to face off a huge and vastly superior Persian army, turned on each other in a brutal and prolonged tussle known as the Peloponnesian War. Shared cultures and values had no place in that war, the priorities of the city state came first.

You will find no greater contrast between city states than that of Athens and Sparta in the fifth century BCE. Athens was a democracy where a number of key positions were decided by lot from the populace, where the people voted on every decision and voted in their fellow citizens to certain public positions; anybody could hold power for at least a short time in Athens. Sparta was a monarchy, a totalitarian state that controlled every aspect of its citizens' lives based on a series of centuries-old laws devised by a man who likely never existed.

Greece, therefore, in terms of this book is less a geographical location and more of an umbrella term for these very different city states that nevertheless had some things in common that on occasions (rare occasions) bound them together.

What do we mean by ancient Greece?

The history of Greek civilisation begins on the island of Crete with the people who historians call the Minoans. I say 'who historians call' because we genuinely have no idea how the people who flourished on Crete between 2000 and 1500 BCE, building fabulous palaces with colourful frescoes and trading goods across the regions of the Mediterranean, referred to themselves.

Minoan was suggested by a British archaeologist working on the island called Arthur Evans. It was the first of many suggestions that Arthur Evans (later Sir Arthur Evans) would put confidently forward about this ancient Cretan civilisation. Evans' Minoan society was a peaceful one in sharp contrast to the times that Evans was living through; an endlessly divided Europe constantly at battle with one another for supremacy. It was also, according to Evans, a matriarchal society, which would make it unique not only in its own era but in every era that followed it.

Evans' guesses, deductions and downright inventions about Minoan culture were the least of it, he also took to physically reconstructing the site. Much of what you will see today at Knossos and marvel at was not built by the Minoans at all but rather by Arthur Evans' crew in the twentieth century. Many of the colourful frescoes attributed to the Minoans were pieced together by Evans' team, often from different parts of what he had determined was a palace (nowadays modern archaeologists think it to be more likely an administrative or religious building)[2] and put together to form an image that never was.

Image 3 shows what purports to be a Terracotta bridge-spouted jar found at Knossos and dating to the middle period of Minoan civilisation around 1900–1600 BCE and a fabulous item it is too. Before you start to verbalise how amazing it is that such an ordinary everyday object should survive intact for 3,000 years and in such good condition too, I'd advise you to take a closer look at the image. Take a real close look and you'll spot the fragments of the original pot around which has been made an entirely new vessel.

The Metropolitan Museum of Art is extremely keen to distance itself from a debate it wants no part of. 'This vase was restored at the Ashmolean Museum, Oxford, before it entered the Museum's collection,' it states on its website.

Minoan comes from the legendary King Minos of Crete, who was the king whose wife had an affair with a bull and whose method of dealing with the monstrous offspring of this adulterous liaison was to build a big labyrinth for the darling half-bull/half-man to play in. Naturally Arthur Evans believed he had discovered this labyrinth too, based on scant evidence and an overly active imagination.

Evans, pioneer of archaeology as he undoubtedly was, serves as a warning of the dangers of viewing the past through the lenses of the present or, in the case of Evans, the lenses of the present and an over-enthused love of Greek mythology. Although to be fair to Evans, recently scholars have looked to re-evaluate his legacy and findings, and concluded that, however he came about his conclusions on the Minoans, he wasn't completely wrong.

After the whoever-the-hell-they-were-but-we'll-call-them-Minoans came the Mycenaeans. The Mycenaeans did their flourishing on mainland Greece in the so-called Bronze Age between 1750 BCE and 1050 BCE, with a key centre of power being the city of Mycenae in Greece's Peloponnese region, hence the name because, as with the Minoans, we don't know what they called themselves. Later Greeks believed that the Mycenaean period was the time during which the heroes that made up their mythology lived, the likes of King Agamemnon of Mycenae, Hector, Achilles, Odysseus and the whole Trojan War gang. This was their peak, their golden era.

It was a golden era that lasted until 1000 BCE-ish when it suddenly didn't. Whatever it was that killed the golden Mycenaean age, it was big and fast because none of them had time to record what ills were destroying them. Though the Mycenaeans did find time to fortify their cities in a way designed to baffle archaeologists ever since. Although it's tempting to think it could have been a big dragon, because why not in an age that the Greeks believed had a half-man/half-bull rampaging around a maze, historians/killjoys suggest it was likely a series of invasions from the Dorian Greeks who are thought to have come from the mountainous regions of Northern Greece.

After the Dorian invasions it all goes a bit quiet on the civilisation front in what becomes known as the Greek Dark Ages, but in the eighth century BCE, from out of the peat bag of history, some green shoots spout upwards, reaching for the light. These green shots were art, literature and lots and lots of pottery of varying designs. These fashions in pottery painting have proved very helpful to archaeologists in dating stuff,[3] much in the way that luminous fingerless gloves, pixie boots and leg warmers enable us to easily identify photographs of ourselves from the 1980s. From this era, known as the Archaic, we see the formation of these independent and very different city states, none of whom feel any kind of brotherly love or attachment to the city state next door. Indeed, they spend most of their histories engaged in warfare with each other, although they down arms long enough to organise the first Olympic Games in 770 BCE.

One of these multitude of city states, Athens, underwent a transformative period after their speculator victory against the Persians. It is this Athens, of the fifth century BCE, that so inspired the Romantics and many others since. It's in this century that we see a flourishing of thoughts and ideas around humanity. There are vast progressions in the fields of art, politics, maths, science, medicine and theatre that inspire and inform our own culture to this very day. So excited were the Athenians by the ideas that were popping out of every man on the street pretty much every day that they decided to write it all down, dedicate a play to it or else plonk it on a vase. This is very handy for us.

Other city states that didn't have ideas pinging off the furniture are a lot more mysterious and unfathomable in what they thought about sex and sexuality. We will try and fathom what we can, but disclaimer up front, most of our evidence for what the ancient Greeks thought about sex and sexuality comes from Athens and from that golden era, post-Persian wars, that lasted from 480 to 404 BCE. We shall be dipping our toes into the Greece that existed before that era and also Greece under the Roman Empire, which is two whole millennia worth of history. The honest response to the question, what do we mean by ancient Greece, is that we mean predominantly fifth-century BCE Athens because that is where our evidence comes from.

How much can we really know about a society's views on such a private matter as sex and sexuality from such a distance in time?

It is true that we very much hindered in our quest to understanding sex and sexuality in ancient Greece by the nature of the sources available to us, particularly literary sources. As noted, the majority of these come from one place, Athens, during one era, the fifth century BCE, but these sources come with another bias: they are all written by men (with the odd exception, hello poetess Sappho) and generally wealthy men of the elite class.

This matters, it matters a lot. There are a lot of missing voices, such as women, slaves and non-citizens. These people collectively far outnumbered the class of our sources, but we can only see them through their eyes. This has led to a lot of fierce debate, over the position of women in Greek society, for example. Are the women in Greek tragedy as depicted by male playwrights a representation of real women of the era? Can philosophical discussions on the nature of women by men tell us anything about what ancient Greek women felt about their lives? Can we really reconstruct and truly understand the beliefs of an entire society on sexuality if we only are able to access the views of such a small, homogenous sample of that society?

The answer to all these questions is probably not (unless you are Sir Arthur Evans and you just make it all up). But along the way we shall determine what we can from what we have been given and uncover way more than you probably ever wished to know about the ancient Greek male mind.

Finally, I want to lob a couple of words at you that will prove useful in our journey through ancient Greece. First up is the word *polis or poleis* as the plural. *Polis* can be used as a snappier and shorter way of saying city state, it refers to the administrative centre of a city and the surrounding area. However, it's also used to refer to the citizen body of that city and the surrounding area also. That that two are interchangeable tells you something already about the nature of the relationship between the ancient Greeks and the state. To us the state is often a distant mysterious and unfathomable creature with strange rules that it compels us to follow and a maddening labyrinth of procedures. In ancient Greece, particularly in democratic Athens, the people were the state.

In Athens the citizens of the city were chosen by lot to serve as officials on a yearly basis, they served as jurors in the law courts, and they were compelled to partake in every vote held on the running of their homeland. There was no unfathomable, unmovable cliff wall of the state against the people, the people were the state.

This changes how we see the laws introduced on issues that touch our topic of sex and sexuality, because we aren't looking at a state that is imposing its idea of what morality is on its citizens, the citizens themselves are creating these laws or at least voting on them.

The second word I'm going to throw at you is *oikos.* This is sometimes translated as family but it encompasses both the people of the family and the property they collectively own. The two most important relationships in ancient Greece are with your *polis* and your *oikos*, as we shall see repeatedly through this book.

But there's also some other important Greek words we are going to need to know to unpick the complexities of sex and sexuality in ancient Greece and they revolve around love.

The language of love

In the English language, the word 'love' is bandied about with an incontinence that devalues and blurs its underlying meaning. Take the seemingly simple statement, 'I love my wife and children.' This singular use of the word is describing two different forms of love; one that involves physical attraction, desire and sexual intercourse and the other that most definitely should not. We intrinsically understand the distinction between those two different kinds of love, much as we understand the distinction between a stated love of a boy band, a TV show, a pet hamster and a steaming hot cup of tea in the morning.

The ancient Greeks were much better than the British at distinguishing these different types of love because they had the words to do so. There was *eros*, which is where our word erotic derives from. *Eros* to the ancient Greeks was the most extreme form of love, an overwhelming passion and desire towards another person. The type of love that propels romance novels and populates the world: boyfriend/girlfriend kind of love. Although with one important difference: this love only flowed in one direction, you could be desired and passionately wanted as the object of *eros* or you could be desiring and passionately wanting as the one inflicted with *eros*, there was no mutual *eros*. *Eros* wasn't always necessarily a positive emotion. *Eros* had its dark side, as we shall explore later in this book.

Whereas *eros* was an all-encompassing emotion that could bring both extreme highs and lows on those afflicted with it, *agape* was a much milder form of love. *Agape* was the kind of love a parent might feel for a child who has come home with a particularly good school report or performed bravely on the field of battle. It's the sort of love that your dog displays with tail-wagging joy when you arrive home from work. It pops up all over the Christian New Testament where it is translated as beloved, as in the 'Dearly beloved,' that begins a sermon or Christ's feelings towards his disciples, his beloved followers. It's affection rather than desire.

There's also *pothos*, which is somewhat like *eros* in that it means to yearn/desire but this is a yearning/desire that is not to be fulfilled. A longing for someone or something that is to remain always a longing. A hopeless form of love that causes a permanent hole in your heart, unrequited love as we would say.

Himeros is that sudden rush of emotion that overwhelms when eyes are first laid on another, love at first sight or captivation as it sometimes gets translated. Like *eros*, *himeros* can have darker connotations and can be linked to the emotions experienced by a would-be rapist as well as one with nobler intentions.

These words for love were personified in Greek mythology, demonstrating a richness to them that is not always evident when used in text. That the Greeks had so many words for love demonstrates its importance to them, which is interesting because it was a society where marriages were arranged for the good of the *oikos*, whether there were any feelings of love between the prospective bride and groom was irrelevant. We are going to find love in some unexpected places in ancient Greece, places that don't correspond to the values and morals of the society we live in today, places that are going to make you feel distinctly uncomfortable.

Part II

Men

Chapter 2

The Body Beautiful

In the fifth century BCE, a sculptor by the name of Polykleitos completed his latest statue, a work known as the *Doryphoros*, or the spear carrier in English. It depicts a young man in the absolute peak of physical fitness; he stands nude, one arm hanging by his side, the other arm lifted slightly. His expression is one of complete sereness, he knows not where his clothes have gone, nor does he care. If I had to describe the *Doryphoros* in one word that word would be 'phwoar', followed by a low whistle whilst fanning myself. He is gorgeous.

I am not alone in thinking this, his creator Polykleitos thought so too. So gorgeous was the *Doryphoros* that Polykleitos felt it crucially important to record his proportions for posterity so that everyone else could produce their own phwoar-worthy statues. Polykleitos' work has sadly been lost to us, but from other sources we can reconstruct some of what it likely said, although not the exact numbers that make the perfect man statue.

Bodily perfection was not only achievable aesthetically in art, it was also achievable in real life too. Second-century CE philosopher Philostratus, who did have access to Polykleitos' numbers, translates what made the perfect marble representation of a man to the fleshy, breathing, wandering-about-a-street-near-you actual man.

> The characteristics of the parts of the body are also to be considered as in sculpture, as follows: the ankle should agree in its measurements with the wrist, the forearm should correspond with the calf and the upper arm with the thigh, the buttock with the shoulder ... for the whole body should be well proportioned to all these other parts.[1]

The fifth-century BCE comic playwright Aristophanes provides us with a helpful checklist of those other attributes aside from proportionality that made up the ideal Greek man's body.

> If you listen and do what I say;
> You'll eternally have:
> A radiant chest, skin that is bright
> Shoulders quite grand, but just a wee tongue
> A sturdy great bum and a miniscule dick.[2]

Which almost perfectly describes the *Doryphoros* and the rows of similarly sturdy bums that line the rooms of any modern museum with an ancient Greek collection.

Aristophanes also helpfully lists what the opposite, an unattractive body looks like:

> Anaemic white skin, shoulders too light
> A chest that's too thin with a tongue that's too long
> A lean upper thigh and a long thing to tweak.[3]

Yes, you read that right, big penises are not considered an attractive or desirable thing to have dangling between your thighs in ancient Greece. A big penis was considered coarse and ugly, a sign of a barbarism and lack of control.

This lack of discipline, self-control and civilised behaviour is personified by the satyrs. Satyrs are mythological creatures depicted with the legs and tail of a horse, pointed ears and permanently erect large penises. You'll find endless images on Greek crockery depicting the antics of satyrs which are linked to the wild/uncontrollable lusts that their large penises exert on them. These include bothering nymphs (see Image 5), animals, wineskins, vases and each other. Satyrs will shag anything.

The perfect Greek male in comparison, as depicted on Greek vases, stands proudly naked with his flaccid, tiny wiener, just as the *Doryphoros* does. Nobody asks ancient Greek women what they think about the benefits of a small penis; however, Greek women were known to masturbate with leather dildos, which may in fact answer our question for us.

The body on display

The body was far more visible in ancient Greece than it is today. Temples and other public spaces were filled with statues of the gods and heroes all of whom, like the *Doryphoros*, were depicted nude with the perfect physique, small penis and all. But it was not just those in the heavenly sphere who were depicted naked.

The Corpus Vasorum Antiquorum is a huge research project dedicated to cataloguing every piece of Greek pottery that has ever been discovered since the project's inauguration in 1922. There is rather a lot of surviving Greek pottery, as demonstrated by the size of the project's database, which currently holds around 100,000 records. You don't have to spend long searching through this database before you inevitably stumble across a scene in which ordinary non-heroic, non-divine Greek men are depicted completely starkers.

I started my search under A with agriculture as the topic and the very first image I came across was of two ancient Greek men leading two oxen tethered to ploughs completely naked (the farmers, that is, although the oxen I suppose are also naked).

This frequent depiction of nudity can mess with our twenty-first-century (filthy) minds. Are those two naked young men depicted smiling and facing each other on a vase about to throw themselves into each other's arms and hit the floor for some passionate lovemaking? Or are they about to hit the floor and attempt to gouge each other's eyes out in a wrestling match? Disappointingly, it's likely to be the latter.

Greek men are depicted doing a lot of things naked together that is quite bewildering to us. Check out Image 6, where we find a man hanging out with his horse; now unless he has extremely tiny pants on, he is grooming his horse completely starkers. I really hope he doesn't ride that horse starkers too, because the chafing would be awful. I give the exact same advice to the two young men in Image 7, who look like they are off for a bit of broke back riding. The naked young man in Image 8 has a decision to make, is he going to javelin practice or is he going to smash those rocks apart his father asked him to do using that that pickaxe? Decisions, decisions… Although he appears to have freed himself from deciding what outfit he's going wear that day, which is something to be said for public nudity, you don't half leave the house quicker on a big night out. Image 9 depicts an Athenian festival dedicated to the god Hephaistos. You have to admire the courage of the men who dare to not only escort what appears to be a not terribly cooperative bull, with the most sensitive part of their bodies fully exposed to bull rage, but also presumably to perform the sacrifice with a very sharp knife that could so easily be knocked into a different trajectory by the unhappy animal.

The question is, and it is one we will ask again and again, how much of the imagery found on Greek pottery is an accurate representation of real life? In this instance, the question we must ask ourselves is did the ancient Greeks really practise wide-scale nudism whilst undertaking everyday tasks?

I think we can conclude probably not, due to the practical reasons mentioned above, chafing and the like. However, it says quite a lot about ancient Greeks that this is how they chose to be represented in art and this is the art they chose to purchase to display in their homes. We are circling back to the Doryphoros and the body beautiful. The Greeks appreciated beauty, they marvelled at its representation by the superstar sculptors of their day. To truly appreciate the beauty of the body and the skill of the artist, one had to see it all.

The place to be seen (naked, naturally)

The Greeks may not have been as naked as their art would have us believe but there is one activity that Greek men definitely did naked together: exercising. This is something that seems to creep in as the norm shortly before the Classical period of Greek history (the fifth and fourth centuries BCE up to Alexander the Great's conquests in 335 BCE) because our writers from this period are sure it's a modern thing, even if none of them can remember the exact moment that they all decided to fling off their clothes for institutionalised nudism.

Historian Thucydides is sure that it was Sparta that started this nude exercising trend, saying that 'the Spartans were the first to bare their bodies and after stripping openly to anoint themselves with oil when they engaged in athletic exercises'.[4] Whereas Isidorus puts this naked innovation as the consequence of an unfortunate wardrobe malfunction during an Athenian foot race when a runner was tripped up by his own baggy shorts. Apparently so grievous a happening was this that the official in charge of the race, determined to prevent such a misfortune ever reoccurring, declared that all Athenians should henceforth exercise in the nude.

Now it is true that the ancient Greeks take sport very seriously, as we shall shortly be discovering, but this tale reeks of implausibility. Most likely it is a hastily cobbled together claim on behalf of the Athenian polis that it was they who invented nude exercising and not the Spartans nor the Megarans nor any of the other city states who seem very keen to get credited with this innovation.

That city states' clamber to get the credit for introducing nude exercising is quite telling. This is not a private pastime, but rather one that comes with a decree from the state and a general agreement from the people that nudity was both preferable and required whilst exercising. As Plato says, 'It was not so long ago it seemed shameful and ridiculous to the Greeks to see men naked. But I suppose that when it became clear to those that used these practices that to uncover all such things is better than to hide them then what's ridiculous to the eyes disappeared in the light of what is best.'[5]

You'll remember earlier in this chapter Aristophanes' description of an unattractive man as having anaemic skin. Proper Greek men were tanned because their naked bodies were fully exposed to the sun when they exercised. A pale body showed that they had not been doing their civic duty. A point that is well made by Spartan king, Agesilaus, who

> gave orders to his heralds that the barbarians that were captured by the Greek raiding parties should be exposed for sale naked. Thus the soldiers, seeing that these men were white-skinned because they were never without their clothing and soft and unused to toil because they always rode around in carriages, came to the conclusion that the war would be in no way different from having to fight with women.[6]

The place where ancient Greek men exercised their way to fully toned and tanned was the gymnasium. Another of those Greek-invented words, gymnasium translates as a place of nakedness, just so there's no misunderstanding as to dress code. These places of nakedness occupy a special space in ancient Greece, they are not places you force yourself to go to for the number of weeks your new year resolve holds, hating every minute of your time there. Gyms in ancient Greece were astonishingly filled with people who wanted to be there, socialising with their fellow citizens. They were the place where men gathered together and hung out, balls out, covered in oil.

The oil was olive oil that the Greeks slathered over their naked bodies and later scraped off along with the sweat and dirt accumulated during their workout with an instrument called a strigil (see Image 11). According to the first-century CE Roman writer Pliny the Elder, the fittest athlete could make a decent profit off their skin gunk, presumably from people who hoped after using it themselves they too would wake up the next morning with pecs to die for. 'The Greeks, progenitors of all vices, have diverted the use of olive oil to serve the ends of luxury by making it available in gymnasia. It is known that those in charge of gymnasia have sold oil that has been scraped off bodies for 80,0000 sesterces.'[7] Eighty thousand sesterces is a ludicrous amount of money. To give you an idea of how ludicrous it is, the annual wage of a soldier in Pliny's era was around 1,200 sesterces.

The type of physical activity that goes on in the gym includes athletic events such as running, javelin and discus throwing but also boxing, wrestling and ball games. These ball games ranged from simple catching to more complicated and brutal-sounding contests. One game known as *episkyros* involved teams of fourteen men trying to push each other over a marked line whilst passing the ball between them; think hardcore rugby.

There was enjoyment to be had in going to the gym aside from exercising and beating up your pals under the guise of sport. The gym was the place to pick up the latest gossip, debate the political fashions of the day and even attend a lecture on the meaning of life at one of the philosophy schools that could be found situated at the gymnasium. Famous philosophers Plato and Aristotle both housed their academies in gyms.

Social spaces, those places where people go to meet their fellow villagers/city dwellers/citizens, tell you a lot about a society. That the pub was the centre of British life until relatively recently tells you a great deal about the British, possibly that we can only converse with each other in a natural fashion with two pints under our belt. For teenagers, a street corner operates as a social space, because they aren't allowed in the pubs or anywhere else vaguely exciting. In other societies the church or other religious building serves as the centre of the community, bringing people together whilst morally improving them. That a place for exercising holds a similar status in bringing people (or rather men, unlike the later Romans and their baths Greek gyms were strictly men only) together in ancient Greece is revealing.

For a start, it puts an emphasis on physical fitness and indeed underlines it several times, possibly with an exclamation mark at the end.

A good body = a good citizen

In the musing of ancient Greeks on the best way to educate children, physical education is given prominence in a way that can only give rise to horror for those of us compelled to play sports we lacked any aptitude for during our school years. Plato ties the physical and the academic forms of education together: 'Am I not right in saying that a good education tends to the improvement of body and mind?' he asks entirely rhetorically, and without pausing for breath goes onto say that, 'growth without exercise of the limbs is the source of endless evils in the body.'[8] Plato determines that if he were running society there would be gymnasia and schools aplenty and these 'will be in the midst of the city'.[9] Attendance will be compulsory for both.

Interestingly, land of Plato schooling also includes dance which we today think of as an expression of art rather than exercise. Plato divides dance into two types, 'the first of them is the more violent, being an expression of joy and triumph after toil and danger; the other is more tranquil symbolizing the continuance and preservation of good.'[10] Which brings forth quite some images in my mind. Spartan dance exercises sound even more bonkers: '[they] danced in the manner in which one would ward off a missile or launch one.'[11]

Plato's not the only one taking an interest in the physical shapes of others, his mentor Socrates greets his presumed friend Epigenes with the less than polite opening line of, 'You look like as if you need exercise.'[12] And then proceeds to harangue poor Epigenes on exactly why him being a bit chubby is so abhorrent. 'For in everything that men do the body is useful, and in all uses of the body it is of great importance to be in as high a state of physical efficiency.'[13] Socrates too links the state of the physical body to the mind: 'Why even in the process of thinking, in which the body seems reduced to a minimum. It is common knowledge that grave mistakes may often be traced to bad health.'[14]

Epigenes' flabby exterior, Socrates gleefully informs him, render him open to the depression, discontent and insanity that a fit body would protect him against. The fit and healthy gain high honours, 'live a pleasanter and better life and leave to their children better means of winning a livelihood',[15] he tells his friend before concluding that Epigenes is a disgrace to treat his body so carelessly.

Xenophon does not record Epigenes' response to this dressing down, which is a pity because we left forever hanging as to whether Epigenes took Socrates' words as true wisdom and was henceforth a total gym bunny, or whether he defended himself by pointing out that his accuser was hardly a specimen of physical perfection either. Our sources make mention of Socrates' snub nose, his projecting eyes and his general resemblance to a satyr. Satyrs are certainly no *Doryphoros*, they are depicted as somewhat chubby and squat. Which I hope is behind the Socrates comparison, as opposed to him walking around Athens with hairy horse legs and a permanent erection, make your own minds up as to their similarity by comparing Images 13 and 14. Nor does Xenophon record whether Epigenes took Socrates out with a single punch and then departed on his chubby legs, whistling happily to himself whilst taking a bite out of the ancient Greek equivalent of a doughnut.

It should be noted that Epigenes is not the only man picked on by Socrates for his failings. Socrates is a man who is constantly questioning everything and everybody and he does so in public, it's his philosophical quirk. Jean-Paul Sartre had a pipe, Freud had a couch and a sex obsession, Socrates was annoying. Socrates was aware how annoying he was, during the trial that would ultimately lead to his death he describes himself as a gadfly, a small insect that nips at livestock but is of no real harm to them.

Chapter 3

The Ultimate Perfection: Athletes

Socrates was not alone in butting his nose into other people's physical fitness, we've seen it before with Plato who, given the chance to install his own state, would have insisted upon everybody reaching physical perfection. This emphasis on physical fitness and exercise was one that inspired another philosopher, again Greek, again Athenian but living in an Athens that was separated from Socrates and Plato by 600 years. His name was Philostratus and he was to go further than any of his predecessors in linking exercise and philosophy.

Obtaining perfection

One day in the third century CE, the philosopher Philostratus finished writing his latest biography of a fellow philosopher we've never heard of and looked up at the world he lived in: he did not like what he saw. What he saw was that 'the athletes of today are inferior to those of earlier times'. The culture had changed from the days of fifth-century BCE Athens where the gymnasium had been the place to hang out, to a society where 'the majority of people are irritated even by lovers of the gymnasium'.[1]

For Philostratus this would not do. Like the Greek philosophers that proceeded him, such as Plato, Philostratus links physical strength and fitness with moral strength and fitness. 'As for athletic training we assert that is a form of wisdom.'[2] But he did not believe that the people of his own day were inferior to those Greeks he so admired from the past. At the centre of his philosophy was that nature was eternal, 'for she still produces men who are spirited and well-formed and quick witted, these are all natural attributes.'[3] No, what had gone wrong in Philostratus' time was the regular and vigorous training his forefathers had undertaken as a standard part of their average day had been all but abandoned by the third century CE. They'd gone soft, abandoning the gymnasium culture of their Greek forefathers for the bathhouse culture of the Romans.

For Philostratus there was more to becoming buff than an hour spent weightlifting or running. The true athlete needed the expertise of a specialised trainer, or *paidotribe*. Something, that again, Philostratus believed was sorely lacking in his times. 'Cleansing the humours and removing excess from the body and smoothing dried-up flesh and fattening or transforming or warming some parts of the body, all of these belong to the wisdom of the trainer.'[4]

What does Philostratus' perfect trainer and dispenser of physical wisdom do to create the perfect athlete like those of the glorious past? Firstly, according to Philostratus, he needed to specialise, a trainer of wrestlers is inexpert in the training of runners and vice versa. Transferable skills is not a term our philosopher gives any credence to. Secondly Philostratus' trainer requires expertise in physiognomy.

Physiognomy according to the encyclopaedia Britannica is 'the study of the systematic correspondence of psychological characteristics to facial features or body structure'. The size of your ears or hands or feet, the distance between your eyes, the bumps and ridges on your skull could all be used to determine what type of person you are. These are all measurable things which makes it feel a bit more sciency than say palm reading, although there really isn't much difference between the two in terms of repeatable results and accuracy of any sort.

Behind physiognomy is the idea that facial features denote positive characteristics or negative characteristics, you can probably see where this is headed already. Once you start categorising features and their corresponding attributes you can then apply them wholesale to the population. You might begin with trying to identify a 'criminal' type based on hundreds of photographs of prisoners, with the noble intent on solving the high crime rate in Victorian London but it's less of a leap and more of a casual step forwards to fall into profiling and categorising the features of various racial groups as being positive or negative. We all know where that leads to.

Philostratus' trainer 'should know all the signs of character in the eyes by which are revealed lazy people, impetuous people and in active people and those people who are less capable of endurance and lacking in self-control'.[5] Although one would think a two-hour gym session would just as easily separate the lazy and inactive than spending years studying eye patterns. Body wise, Philostratus is looking for that *Doryphoros* symmetry of proportion in all the would-be athletes' bodies.

But it was not good enough to have the perfect body and temperament of an athlete, you also had to have the correct background: 'let the trainer approach the boy athlete and examine him first of all with reference to his parents, considering whether they were young when they were married and in excellent condition and free from illness.'[6] The offspring of older parents are detectable because their skin is delicate and their collarbones are hollowed out, Philostratus tells us before going to inform us that they are also sluggish, do not colour when they exercise and are incapable of picking anything up without needing a rest afterwards.

Having selected their protégé, the trainer's job seems to involve a lot of steering his ward away from pursuits incompatible with training. Sensible things such as not overeating nor excessively drinking, having energy-sapping sex and sunbathing. Although Philostratus puts a caveat on that last one, 'ignorant' sunbathing is what he objects to because everyone knows that 'the kinds of sunshine that accompany the north wind and come on windless days are clean and healthily sunny … but those that accompany the south wind or come on overcast days are most and burn excessively and are liable to enfeeble those in training.'[7] To which we add metrology to the trainer's skillset alongside physiognomy and genealogy.

Having selected the perfect protégé from a good study of his features, the features of his parents and steered him away from anything fun that might use up valuable energy, and put him through a vigorous series of exercises over a prolonged period, the trainer could now enter his ward into an athletic competition. Which sounds like a positive thing, right? The chance for the protégé to make his trainer proud and prove himself worthy. But being an elite athlete comes with risks attached, as Philostratus earlier hints at. 'But if someone has a break or a flesh wound or clouding of his eyes or a dislocation of one of his limbs, then he needs to be taken to the doctor for the art of the athletic trainer does not concern itself with problems of this kind.'[8] Greek sport was dangerous, there was a high chance of injury and some of those injuries could come from your own trainer.

Eryxias, the trainer of a *pankratiast* (the *pankration* was a sport that mixed elements of boxing, wrestling and the sort of brutal punishment beatings you hear about happening in prisons), seeing his protégé flagging, 'inspired him with a desire for death, by shouting from the sidelines, "What a fine funeral shroud not to give up at Olympia."'[9] Eryxias was clearly a skilled trainer because he inspired such a desire for death in his protégé that the protégé did actually die during this bout. I suppose we could mark this down as a death by proxy but Philostratus has another more straightforward case of death by trainer.

The story told is of a dubious origin, which even Philostratus recognises, opening with the telling, 'but there are some who say…'[10] The some that say tell of an athlete who was killed at Olympia by his strigil-wielding trainer, 'as punishment for not exercising endurance in his pursuit of victory'.[11] You might want to flick to Image 11 to remind yourself what a strigil looks like. They are bent at the end which would make them a poor weapon for stabbing someone with, although this one had been especially sharpened, we are told, which still doesn't make it a good stabbing implement. Perhaps it was used to beat the athlete to death with. Our exercise guru Philostratus is fully onboard with this murder. 'Let the strigil be the word against worthless athletes!'[12] he declares, adding, 'let the trainer at Olympia rank in some respects above the father.' You wouldn't want Philostratus as your personal trainer, he'd happily jog you to death.

There is no mention of either trainer being punished themselves for causing the death of the young man they had spent hours of their lives moulding into an elite athlete, far from it, Philostratus praises the murderer. Which is a small taster for what was the true nature of ancient Greek sport and competitions. Nobody was shaking hands at the end of a match, swapping shirts and praising the skill of their opponents in ancient Greek sports. There wasn't even the equivalent of a silver or bronze medal; in Greece you were the winner or you were one of many losers. It's time to meet the winners.

Heroes in the flesh

In a society that placed such emphasis on physical exercise and perfection of body it is not surprising that athletes were elevated to the rank of heroes and most importantly winners. The word athlete translates as 'one who is competing for a prize'. Athletes were the supreme prize winners, rewarded and lionised for the efforts they put into achieving perfection. They toured Greece taking part in competition after competition. The sheer number of competitions is highlighted by Emperor Nero winning an incredible 1,808 first prizes during his eighteen-month tour of Greece in the 60s CE.

Yes, Nero was taking part in multiple events in a single competition and yes, the Greeks probably awarded him more prizes than were usually on offer to competitors who didn't have the advantage of unlimited power over a large chunk of the known world. However, at least Nero took part in these competitions in the flesh because previously, 'the cities in which it was the custom to hold contests in music had adopted the rule of sending all the lyric prizes to him'.[13] Which is quite an addition to the 'how to suck up to an emperor at minimal cost for the greatest of benefits' cheat sheet.

So delighted was Nero by these prizes he kept winning without needing even to get out of bed, let alone write a poem to enter, he decided to bestow his Imperialness upon the Greek nation. They bloody loved him, he bloody loved them and as a result of that love fest Nero declared somewhat unexpectedly that the Greeks who lived in the province of Achaea need never pay taxes again. Achaea just happened to be where the Isthmus Games were held, which Nero had enthusiastically and very successfully taken part in (possibly requiring another wagon to transport all his prizes back to Rome).

This is a tremendous and awe-inspiring bit of sucking up to the big guy, but Nero's wagonloads of prizes are not so far out there. Theogenes of Thebes, who competed as a *pankratiast* and boxer in the early fifth century BCE, totted up 1,200 or 1,400[14] prizes depending on which historian you choose to believe, admittedly over his entire career rather than a two-year period as Nero had. As a comparison, the man who holds the record as the most decorated athlete in the modern Olympics, American swimmer Michael Phelps, won a career total of only eighty-two medals, sixty-five of them being gold medals. Loser.

It is estimated there were around 300 competitions of varying size and importance held across the Mediterranean by the second century CE.[15] The biggest and most prestigious of these competitions were the Panhellenic Games which were made of up of the Pythian Games, the Nemean

Games, the Isthmian Games and of course the most famous of them all, the Olympic Games.

The Nemean and Isthmian Games took place every two years, and the Delphic and Olympic every four. Of these games the Olympic were the most prestigious and important. So important were they that the Greeks used them to measure time, and you will find references to events occurring during the year of the 76th Olympiad, for example. Although this dating system was to be scuppered by the Emperor Nero's tour of Greece. Nero wasn't prepared to wait around four whole years for the chance to compete in the Olympics, not when the Greeks could reschedule their entire competition cycle especially for him. This was later fixed after Nero's ignoble suicide in 68 CE by the judges of this 211th Olympiad, they declared the whole event void and stripped the emperor of his victories, whilst repaying the bribes they had taken from him for awarding those victories.

Some of the events staged at the Panhellenic Games will be familiar to us from the modern Olympic Games; there were running races, discus and javelin throwing, wrestling and boxing. Equestrian events were included such as horse racing and chariot racing. Other events are more novel, there was the *pankration* which was a brutal mix of boxing and wrestling, and the hoplite race, both of which we will take a deeper look at later in this chapter.

The Pythian Games, alongside the usual sporting events, also held music and poetry competitions, as did the Nemean and Isthmian Games. It was the Olympics only that exclusively concentrated on the physical sports, although again it made an exception for the Emperor Nero, who insisted they be included for the first time in the 800-year history of the Olympics purely so he could enter and win more prizes. Which is something we'd all do given unlimited power.

That music and poetry were just as much a part of the Panhellenic Games (excepting the Olympics) as the discus or the running sprints links back to Plato and co. and the links they made between mental and physical exercise. Today we think of them as two quite distinct categories: art and sport. To the ancient Greeks they were far more intertwined.

As with the non-professional regulars at the gymnasium, the professional athlete competed naked, the exceptions to this rule being chariot racing and the artistic, non-sporting competitions. Because of this nudity, the Olympics and the other Panhellenic Games were strictly men only, no women were allowed to participate or spectate. Although some people dispute this and say that it was only married women who were banned from being spectators, unmarried girls being free to ogle away. That there are countering views to this tells you one thing, women barely get a mention in any of the sources we have relating to the games.

Where women do get a mention is surprisingly in the lists of Olympic winners, because the victors of the equestrian events were not the jockeys speeding their horse across the finish line but rather the owners of the winning horse. Women could and did own horses.

Knyiska, the daughter of a Spartan king, is listed as an Olympic champion in the four-horse chariot race and a statue dedicated to her victories in two Olympiads.

As well as competing naked, the athletes would also cover themselves in olive oil for reasons which have become obscure. Did the rubbing of the oil into the flesh warm up the muscles suitably for competition? Or was the oil merely aesthetic, a way of showing off those male bodies to perfection, glistening as the oil reflected the bright sun? Or was it of more practical use aiding the athlete to scrape off the dirt and sweat from his body post competition using his strigil?

Similarly mysterious in its benefits was the practice of infibulation. We see infibulation portrayed on pottery from the era where it looks distinctly like the posed athletes have tied a little bow round their penises, which would be delightful and something I would encourage every man to do for their lady or man friend, because it makes for a lovely surprise and cheers up the appearance of male genitalia. Disappointingly, this is not what infibulation is. Rather than an eye-pleasing adornment to the penis, infibulation is the tying down of the foreskin with string over the glans (the tip of the penis), a practice that has generated over the centuries many, many paragraphs in academic papers and books all seeking to answer the same question, why in Zeus' golden thunderbolt would you want to do that? And then, how do you do that?

Circumcision was not practised in ancient Greece; it was thought of as abhorrent. In a society where public nudity was a thing, we might therefore expect to see an emphasis on displaying your fully intact tackle in as full a form as possible. However, infibulation was not widely practised in ancient Greece and appears to be restricted to the region of Attica, whose dominant city was Athens. From surviving images, it also appears restricted to those participating in athletics or exercising in the gym.

That we only find infibulation linked to sport suggests that it was thought to be of benefit to athletes. Some depictions of infibulation show the string wound round the penis serving to tuck it in as well as hold down the foreskin which would suggest that maybe it increased performance, the athlete rendered more aerodynamic without that thing flopping between his legs the whole time and make running more comfortable for him. Or perhaps it served to protect the penis and foreskin in close-quarter events like wrestling where its delicate sensitivities could be used against its owner. Though if this was the case you would expect it to be taken up by all athletes, for which of them wasn't looking for anything that might give them an advantage, but it isn't.

Which leaves us with what explanation for infibulation? I suspect that we have to look back at those Athenian ideas of beauty that influenced the carving of the swoonsome *Doryphoros* and the countless clones that followed him, all of them sporting neat, tidy and tiny penises. Sporting endeavours ruined that beauty, they drew attention to the penis flopping about ungainly between thighs. Best to tie it up in a manner that was referred to by other Greeks as a dog leash to preserve the dignity, beauty and perfection of the athletic body.

The ultimate prize

The Panhellenic Games were what every athlete and poet wanted to triumph at. They were the pinnacle of your career and immortality followed a victory. Philostratus, who is writing in the second and third centuries CE, reels off a list of prize-winning athletes. 'Milo, Hipposthenes, Poulydamas and Promachus.'[16] That he reels off these names without any further explanation or description of their victories shows how famous these athletes were, which is quite something given Milo lived a cool 800 years before Philostratus is writing, as did Hipposthenes. Poulydamas and Promachus won their victories in the fifth century BCE, 600 years prior. I doubt there are many of us who could reel off any more than a half a handful of Olympics winners from the 1920s and 30s, if any at all, and that's only a hundred years ago. The Greeks were familiar with athletes that pre-dated them by a millennium.

One reason why Philostratus can casually reel off his list of athletic victors is that there were physical reminders of them that still stood in his day. At Olympia, site of the Olympic Games, it was standard to erect statues of the victors of individual games. These statues are exhaustively listed in the work of Pausanias, a second-century CE Greek who produced a guidebook to Greece for the discerning tourist, the discerning tourist who likes to read. Pausanias' *Guide to Greece* is a whopper of a book; its current publisher Penguin Classics publishes it as two volumes, each over 500 pages long. The most recent Lonely Planet guide to Greece limits itself to a single volume of 600-odd pages and it has 2,000 years more of historical sites to suggest visiting than Pausanias had. I think we can say Pausanias was a thorough travel writer.

Thorough he may have been, but such were the numbers of statues dedicated to Olympic victors that even he must limit himself on how many he is going to include in his book. 'Those only will be mentioned who themselves gained some distinction, or whose statues happened to be better made than others,'[17] he decides. Nevertheless, I counted seventy-one statues Pausanias writes about, before I gave up counting halfway through the chapter on the basis I really, really needed a cup of tea and that I'd ceased to care about any more athletes and their amazing accomplishments.

Pausanias was not alone in undertaking such a detailed task. Fourth-century BCE philosopher Aristotle compiled a full list of Olympic victors, again showing how to the Greeks fitness of mind and body were equal. Today we tend to categorise people as either sporty or intellectual and determine that you follow one path or the other. Respect for the intelligence of the elite sportsperson in our society is restricted to gaining a decent score on the BBC quiz show *A Question of Sport*. Completely unfairly the default assumption is that sportspeople, particularly footballers, are on the dim side. Similarly, the intellectual is assumed to be rubbish at sport, again completely unfairly. For all we know, Richard Dawkins is ace at five-a-side football and Wayne Rooney is an avid reader of Tolstoy, facts we would never discover if true, because no journalist or feature writer is ever going to pose the questions that would reveal them.

On some of these statues Pausanias has little information to impart, others he has a raft of stories to relate on. There is Sostratus, who 'used to grip his antagonist by the fingers and bend them and would not let go until he saw his opponent had given in'.[18] Ouch. Although Sostratus was not alone in this tactic, it appears. The wrestler 'Leontiscus did not know how to throw his opponents, but won by bending their fingers.'[19] There is Pulydamos, who was 'the tallest of all men who except those called heroes and other mortal race that may have existed before the heroes'.[20] And tragically, the wrestler Chilon, who won two crowns at Olympia, one at Delphi, four at Isthmus and three at the Nemean Games, only to be defeated on the battlefield where he met his death.

The most famous athlete both Philostratus and Pausanias, and many others, mention is Milo of Croton. Croton was a Greek settlement in Southern Italy and Milo the wrestler was their most famous son. In a career spanning decades, Milo totted up five wins in five Olympic Games, which puts him level with British rower Steve Redgrave, who won five gold medals at five consecutive Olympic Games from 1984 to 2000 and, fittingly, Greco-Roman wrestler Mijan Lopez, who also has five gold medals from five consecutive games from 2008 to 2024.[21]

However, when Milo turned up for his sixth Olympics, he won by default because nobody else turned up to fight him. He was a legend, as Pausanias tells his audience: 'They say too, that Milo carried his own statue into the Altis.'[22] The Altis being the sanctuary of the gods where all the statues of the Olympic heroes were erected and to where Milo carried the bronze statue of himself. Milo did not limit his amazing displays of strength to Olympia and the sites of the other Panhellenic Games, he was quite happy to show them off out of competition too. There was the time he carried a bull, yes, a fully grown bull, on his shoulders, a feat impressive enough on its own but Milo goes further than mere bull lifting and carrying, he killed the bull singlehandedly and then butchered and ate it whole in a single day. (Disclaimer: We strongly advise readers against any attempts to emulate any of Milo's stunts. A full-grown bull weighs between 500 and 1,000 kg, 340 kg approximately of that weight is edible meat.)

Three hundred and forty kilograms is a hell of a lot of beefburgers or steak Dianes. In fact, it's equivalent to nearly 3,000 quarter-pound burgers, which, let's face it, is an impossible number to physically eat in a single day given there are only 1,440 minutes to be had in a day. Milo would have to be eating the equivalent of 2.08 quarter-pound burgers per minute and that's before we even contemplate what that would do to the human digestive system. But that is by the by, Milo was clearly such a specimen of manhood that people were prepared to believe any tales told about him no matter how implausible.

I have an inkling that Milo might well be responsible for the exaggerated embellishments of what was probably a true tale involving some feat of strength and a bull. He certainly wasn't shy of showing off his skills and we find other, more plausible stories about his legendary strength that revolve more realistically, if less dramatically, around fruit. It was said that such was his grip that nobody could take a piece of fruit out of his hand once he had hold of it.

In Pausanias' take on the tale the fruit is a pomegranate, in Pliny the Elder's tale the fruit is different, but the trick is the same: 'when he gripped an apple, nobody could straighten his fingers.'[23] Which strongly suggests a public performance of some sort and a challenge set to be the first person to successfully retrieve the fruit from Milo's grip. Although I'm thinking surely a pomegranate would squish to a pulp in Milo's meaty grip.

Another one of his tricks was to burst a band off his head by inhaling and expanding the veins in his head, which no man has any reason to do beside to show off that he can. Milo was a man who created his own legend and lived it to the full.

It is fitting that the manner of Milo's death should be as legendary and show-offy as the manner of his life, he was never going to be a man who expired quietly after a short illness. His demise came about when he punched a tree in half, got his hands wedged in the split and was eaten alive by wolves. There's a lesson in that tale somewhere about the worthlessness of great feats if there is no one to witness them, about abusing the powers the gods have given you and paying the price, or about how man is nothing compared to nature and that nature will always triumph. Grand themes like that. Although my takeaway is never ever to go wandering around any woodland where you could possibly encounter a wolf. But then I'm from Britain where the most dangerous animal you are ever likely to encounter in a wood is a slightly narked squirrel or a grumpy badger.

What is noticeable about Pausanias' descriptions of the Olympic statues is that for each one the inscription lists which part of Greece or the colonies the athlete had come from. Their fame brought lustre to their hometowns, and they were clearly proud to represent them. Which I guess we shouldn't be surprised at given the fierce competition between the city states and the near-constant warfare between them. It had to make for an edgy atmosphere at Olympia with everyone camped out together for the duration of the games. Surprisingly, astonishingly even, there are no clashes between supporters along the lines of modern football hooliganism recorded. The ideals of the ancient Olympics that each state lay down their arms during the games was rigidly upheld, aided no doubt by the religious element that was as intrinsic a part of the festival as any of the sporting events that took place. Nobody wanted to piss off Zeus by sullying the festival he presided over, not when there was a victory at stake for their guy.

That Pausanias spends quite so much time listing these statues is mostly, one suspects, because he is a thorough chap (he really is) and he has set himself this task of writing an educational guidebook and by the gods above he is going to do that! No Roman tourist pottering around Greece will ever look at a statue, temple, monument and think, 'What the Hades is that?' Not with Pausanias' book in his leather satchel! But he also has to be thinking what will my readers like to some degree, else why leave some statues out as he states? Pausanias' Roman readers, the author deduces, are going to want to know about at least seventy-one Olympic victors, most of whom died hundreds of years before they were born. As you are probably gathering, the Olympics were a big deal, arguably bigger than even the modern Olympics are because the stakes were much, much higher.

The winner takes it all

In July 1988, the delegations of three countries waited with anticipation to hear which of them had won the honour of hosting the most prestigious sporting competition in the world. This is a sporting event with a devoted worldwide television audience of 3.6 billion that during its four-week run would dominate newspaper front pages and conversations in every pub/bar/café/hairdressers on every continent on this planet of ours. This sporting event was the Football World Cup.

In 1988, only six national teams – Uruguay, Italy, Germany, Brazil, Argentina and, yes, England – had held aloft that golden trophy. Along the way the hopes, the dreams, the very hearts of other nations had been squished like a pomegranate in Milo of Croton's hands. The World Cup is one of the few occasions where it is not uncommon, in fact it's expected to see grown men weeping like children who have dropped their ice cream on the dirt floor before getting a first lick. It's a big deal, all right.

In 1988, the three countries vying to host this giant global event were three-times winner Brazil, zero-times winners but enthusiastic participants, Morrocco,[24] and the United States of America, a nation that has never really embraced football, or soccer as they insist on calling it, like the rest of the world has. The viewing figures for the 2022 World Cup final in the USA, a country with a population of 250 million, was a paltry 3.59 million compared with the 42.9 million Brazilian football fans out of a population of 219 million who tuned into the final. Still, it was hoped that staging the World Cup in the USA would maybe increase national interest in a game that the Americans were very meh on.

As you can see from the figures I've quoted for the 2022 World Cup, it clearly didn't, but the 1994 World Cup isn't just infamous for being held in a country largely indifferent to it, it's also infamous for being the scene of an incident that would lead to 27-year-old Andres Escobar being shot multiple times outside a nightclub in Medellin, Colombia.

Escobar would not survive his injuries, nobody could have, not even a fit young athlete like Escobar was. For Andreas Escobar, only one week earlier, had been at the Rose Bowl stadium in Pasadena as part of the Colombia national football team. The match had been versus the hosting nation, the USA, and was the last of the group matches. Both teams needed a win to secure their place in the next round.

Ten minutes into the game, Escobar made a terrible mistake. Trying to pass the ball from an American strike on their goal back to the Colombian goalkeeper, Escobar instead kicked the ball into his own net, putting the opposing team ahead by a goal. It was a lead the USA team consolidated by a further goal in the second half. Although Colombia managed to rally themselves to scoring a goal in the ninetieth minute of the game, it was too little, too late.

For the USA football team, this was a historic moment, it was their first victory in a World Cup game since 1950, a sweet victory made all the sweeter by being on home ground. For Colombia it was a brutal humiliation of an exit. For Escobar it signed his death warrant. Astonishingly, I am not making this up. The reason Escobar was gunned down outside that night club was because of that own goal, a fact his killers made no secret of, yelling out 'GOAL!' as they fired at him.

Newspaper headlines from the time decry it as a senseless killing, and it does seem senseless to us that such a young man should lose his life over a mistake made in what is, passion aside, just a game. It would have made much more sense to the ancient Greeks, they would have seen it as understandable.

'There was a law among the Plataeans … that anyone who was defeated having previously won should be publicly executed.'[25] The Panhellenic Games were a serious and sometimes deadly business. The Plataeans, like Andreas Escobar, faced death back in their homelands but it was not unknown for athletes to be killed during the competition itself.

The victor of the *pankration* event at the 54th Olympiad, which took place in 564 BCE, remained silent and unmoved as the olive wreath crown of victory was placed upon his head and the crowd went nuts cheering all around him. The newly crowned victor, Arrhichion, was stoically silent, not because he'd held such supreme confidence in his abilities that he'd expected to win and felt he'd got merely what was due to him, nor because he'd won at the previous Olympic Games and so it wasn't quite so exciting as his first victory. No, Arrhichion's solemn demeanour and lack of excitement at being crowned an Olympic champion was solely down to the fact that he was dead.

It had been during the final match of the *pankration* that Arrhichion had been held in a lock by his opponent and suffocated in front of a cheering crowd and his trainer, who was shouting out the encouragements around how an Olympic victory was a fine funeral shroud. Arrhichion took his trainer's advice on board and managed to deliver a stunning victory at the very moment of his own earthly defeat. During what would be his very last breath, Arrhichion somehow found the strength to deliver a blow which dislocated his opponent's toe. In agony, the opponent signalled his surrender to the judges, at which point Arrhichion, knowing he had won, carked it. This is presented in our sources as a glorious triumph over circumstance, whilst ignoring the circumstance was a young man suffocating to death in front of hundreds of people who let it happen and the man who had trained and mentored him for years actively encouraging it.

The *pankration* is but one of the sports in which we know of competitors being killed during a match. The word *pankration* translates as 'complete strength' or 'complete victory', and it most certainly was a demonstration of this. Although it involved elements of boxing and wrestling, it was a distinctly different event, an all-out fight whose result was decided only when a competitor signalled that they were unwilling or unable to continue. There were only two rules that we know of; you weren't allowed to bite your opponent, nor were you allowed to gauge out his eyes. Judges were on hand, armed with sticks ready to stop any infringement of these two tactics, but would stand by and allow every other form of violence, including the snapping of fingers and strangulation. It's astonishing that we find repeat Olympic *pankration* champions because the injuries sustained to reach the final had to be profound. We have no equivalent to the *pankration* today, at least nothing legal.

If being suffocated to the cheers of your opponent's fanbase with two judges standing by watching your final moments wasn't horrific enough, the Nemean Games were the scene of the horribly violent death of a boxer.

> Damoxenus with straight fingers struck his opponent under the ribs; and what with the sharpness of his nails and the force of the blow he drove his hand into the other's inside, caught his bowels, and tore them as he pulled them out. Creugas expired on the spot, and the Argives expelled Damoxenus for breaking his agreement by dealing his opponent many blows instead of one. They gave the victory to the dead Creugas, and had a statue of him made in Argos.[26]

I don't think we need to dig down any further into this story. Ick.

The creator of the modern Olympic Games, Pierre de Courbetin, described his vision for the games and their competitors as creating a 'way of life based on the joy of effort, the educational value of good example, social responsibility and respect for universal fundamental ethical principle'.[27] Which is very far removed from Creugas having his bowels ripped out and the routine tactic of finger snapping in the ancient Games.

The ancient Greeks had no notion of sportsmanship, ethical principles (whatever they are) never crossed their minds, all they were concerned about was winning, winning at any cost. There were no silver or bronze medals at the Panhellenic Games, nor any kudos gained for trying your best. You were either the winner or you were a loser. This obsession with winning is very important, even crucial to understanding ancient Greece and why exercise and sport were so central to its society. As is one particular event that took place at the Olympic and other Panhellenic Games: the hoplite race.

The hoplite race was the only running event where the participants did not partake wholly naked, instead they ran dressed in a helmet and metal shin pads and carrying a shield. Shields are ungainly things to run with, especially Greek shields which were designed to be used by an army who fought in formation. In battle these shields, held altogether in a military formation known as a phalanx, protected the shield holder and his buddy to the left of him, such was their size. According to military historians a hoplite shield was around 80–100 centimetres long and could weigh up to 8 kg. This is equivalent to the weight of two newborn babies or a microwave oven (choose your favourite comparison), and along with those bronze shin pads and helmet, these shields added an extra dollop of gruel to a running race. Why it existed as a sport makes sense when you find out what a hoplite was, in fact it makes the brutal competitiveness and violence of ancient sport we have covered in this chapter all make sense; a hoplite was a Greek soldier.

We have reached what is the crux of the Greek obsession with the body beautiful and it is maybe not what you expected, because it's less about beauty and more about brutality, the brutality of war, that is.

Being prepared

There is a reason for all this emphasis on physical fitness, bodily perfection and the hero worship of athletes and it's nothing to do with vanity or an improved ability to score in the sex department (although both of these likely played a part in it). We delved previously into Plato's ideas on the importance of physical education, an education he was all for making compulsory, 'whether their parents like it or not; for they belong to the state more than their parents'.[28] This is the key to understanding everything we have looked at in this chapter.

Athens and many of the other city states did not have a standing army like we do today (the exception being Sparta, who we will look at shortly) or even like the Romans did a few centuries later, their army is composed of the citizen male class. The army that defeated that huge invading Persian army in 480 BCE was not made up of professional soldiers, it was made up of the ordinary citizen men of the city state.

In this context that bonkers Spartan dancing makes more sense, they are aping in dance the launching of missiles as practice for the real thing. Those brutal ball games where two teams pushed at each other? Training for both cooperating in rank with your own team and facing off united against an enemy. Socrates' rant at the flabby Epigenes? A large part of his argument for Epigenes getting his arse down the gym is linked to the necessity of fitness in battle. 'The fit are healthy and strong; and many as a consequence save themselves decorously on the battlefield.'[29] The obsession with winning with no credit given to runners up in the Panhellenic Games? Building mental resilience and determination, for in war there is no runner up, no consolation prize. One side wins, and the other loses. Every city state needed to be the winner.

In Athens every young male citizen, known collectively as *ephebes*, had to undertake two years of military training which marked the transition from childhood into becoming a full member of the *polis*. A young man turned adult could also expect to be called up for further military training alongside his fellow tribe members.[30] Every adult male, of any tribe, could be called up at any time if war should break out.

This was no idle threat. The suspension of war for the Olympic Games is highlighted in ancient sources because it was rare for Greeks to experience peace among themselves. It was imperative that the Greek male citizen kept himself in shape, his life and the lives of his tribe, fellow citizens and his *polis* itself depended on it.

Xenophon recounts how the father of the Persian king, Cyrus, advised him that the best way to manage an army was to allow his troops little leisure time but plenty of time for physical activities. 'What a burden it is to support even one idle man! It is more burdensome to support a whole household in idleness; but the worst burden of all is to support an army in idleness.'[31] If your enemy was making sure their army was in the best physical shape, then the Athenians and other Greek city states sure had to do so as well.

Lurking behind Xenophon's words is the history of past Greek encounters with the Persians. The Greeks working together had successfully repelled King Xerxes' invasion in 480 BCE, but that victory had not come easy, Athens had been destroyed by the rampaging Persians. This was not something that had been forgotten by the Athenians and nor could it be, for the city was awash with physical reminders. Athens had been rebuilt from the rubble the Persians had left behind. They had suffered greatly but they had ultimately triumphed. These new buildings, such as UNESCO World Heritage Site and tourist hotspot, the Parthenon,[32] commemorated this victory.

This was a victory won because of the Greek obsession with sport.

> That wrestling and pankration were devised for their usefulness for warfare is clear first of all from their achievements at Marathon where the battle was fought by the Athenians in such a way that it seemed like a wrestling contest and secondly from the events at Thermopylae where the Spartans when their swords and spears were broken, accomplished much with their bare hands.[33]

The brutality of the *pankration* was perfect training for the brutality of war with a Greek side not afraid of inflicting the greatest physical pain they could. The hoplite race trained men in the practicalities of war, how to hold onto your shield whilst in motion, getting used to moving with speed whilst wearing heavy armour and a vision-restricting helmet.

Chapter 4

Bodily Perfection the Spartan Way

In ancient Athens, as we have seen, the army was made up of the citizen body, hence the emphasis on exercise, physical perfection and the two years of conscripted training every young man undertook, as well as partaking in regular exercises with his fellow citizens. Athens did rather well because of this, becoming the dominant power in Greece and slyly building itself an empire.[1]

This empire building would put Athens at conflict with one of the other dominant city states of the time, Sparta. You'll have heard of Sparta. You'll have heard about those 300 Spartans who held back the massive force of King Xerxes' army at Thermopylae long enough for the rest of the Greeks to organise themselves into the force that would ultimately repel the Persian invaders from Greece. The Battle of Thermopylae has been depicted heroically in the 1962 movie *The 300 Spartans* and completely bonkers in the 2006 movie *300*.

The film *300* portrays King Xerxes as a 7ft tall alien fond of jewellery who talks as if speaking through those voice distorters terrorists used to use to phone in bomb threats. The Persians under Xerxes' command are a bunch of mutant perverts with battle rhinos. I'm told that this is a clever way of helping us understand how truly different the invading army from the East must have appeared to the Greeks of the time. The Spartans in *300* fight in their underpants and shout, 'We are Sparta!' at each other a great many times as they build a defensive wall constructed out of the corpses of Persian soldiers and their battle rhinos. Professional historians have all let slide because none of them have the spare time to compile a list of all the historical inaccuracies in the film *300*. Nobody does.

Accompanying this knowing self-sacrifice for the good of a Greece they'd only just decided existed, Spartans are remembered for their pithy macho one-liners which are helpfully preserved for us by first-century CE biographer Plutarch. When King Leonidas was told, as he arrived to defend Thermopylae, that the Persians had so many arrows they blotted out the sun, an unfazed Leonidas retorted, 'Won't it be nice then if we shall have some shade to fight them in.'[2] When the Persian King Xerxes ordered the Spartans to lay down their weapons, Leonidas' reply was, 'Come and take them.' Then there's this classic one to Philip II of Macedon's grandstanding that if he invaded Laconia (the area of Greece in which Sparta was located) he would turn all the Spartans out, the reply to which was, 'If.' To another letter from Philip issuing demands they simply responded, 'What you wrote about. No.' Which I intend to henceforth use as a reply to any irritating work emails.

This is what is at the heart of Sparta worship and Elon Musk's post on the social media site he owns, X, 'It is remarkable that Sparta had no walls when all other cities did.' A reference to how inconceivable it was that anyone would dare to invade Sparta because of their military prowess. As opposed to a comment on the terrible lack of builders and similarly skilled tradesmen in ancient Sparta, which I think we'd all be more sympathetic towards Sparta about. It's a direct reference to one of Plutarch's compiled Spartan sayings, this one is attributed to King Agis. 'As he was going amongst the walls of the Corinthians and observed that they were high and towering and vast in extent, he said, "What women live in that place."'[3]

Elon isn't alone in expressing admiration for ancient Sparta. The USA has numerous towns named after a city that predates their country by 2,000 years. There are Spartas to be found in Tennessee, New Jersey, Georgia, Kentucky, Louisiana, Missouri, Mississippi, Nebraska, North Carolina, Ohio, Wisconsin and Michigan.

The Sparta located in Michigan has full-on branded itself with the Michigan State University, naming all of its sports teams Spartans. There's the Michigan State University Spartans American Football Team, the Michigan State University Spartans Track and Field Team, the Michigan State University Spartans Baseball Team and on and on it goes all the way to the Michigan State University Spartans Golf Team. I find it particularly hard to imagine a group of ancient Spartans playing a genteel game of golf. Not without the loser being clubbed to death with a putter over the eighteenth hole as a lesson to the others that to be Spartan is to win.

A quick bit of internet research reveals a website dedicated to what are dubbed 'Spartan races'. They are all endurance-style runs, which is not what I would call fun, but apparently enough people do for the company involved to stage six different kinds of races, all with macho names such as the Beast and the Ultra. The ultra-Spartan race is described as 'a 50k trail curse with rugged ascents and 60 demanding obstacles to present a uniquely brutal and physical challenge. It is the ultimate test of endurance and perseverance for the toughest Spartan.'[4] Hmmm. I think I'll pass on that one too.

Sparta, to the twenty-first-century mind, or at least to the twenty-first-century mind who works in advertising and branding, conjures up images of excellence in extreme sport and fitness with a side order of raw masculinity. Elsewhere Paul Cartledge in his book on the Spartans defines the less commercialised Sparta worshipping that the likes of Musk muse on in between making his billions.

> While Athens is justly credited with phenomenal achievements in visual art, architecture, theatre, philosophy and democratic politics, the ideals and traditions of its greatest rival, Sparta, are equally potent and enduring; duty, discipline the nobility of arms in a cause worth dying for, the sacrifice of the individual for the greater good of the community and the triumph of will over seemingly insuperable obstacles.[5]

The Spartan idea of community and the greater good deviates substantially from what Sparta's American admirers might like to believe; for a start this community was compulsory and it demanded all manner of other sacrifices from its citizens besides giving up their lives in a hopeless battle they had not a chance of winning.

The military model to perfection

Whereas Athens had a part-time army of buffed-up citizens who fat-shamed each other into regular gym attendance, Sparta wasn't taking any chances on its citizens freely choosing to keep in shape. 'It was likewise ordered by Law, that every tenth day the young men should shew themselves naked before the *Ephori*; If they were of a solid strong constitution, and melded as it were for exercise, they were commended; but if any limb was found to be soft and tender by reason of fatness accrued by idleness, they were beaten and punished.' Which makes Socrates' jibes seem positively cuddly in comparison.

That Sparta should have a law that stated, 'That no *Lacedemonian* shall be of an unmanly complexion, or of greater weight then is fit for the exercises,'[7] is not terribly surprising because Sparta is big on laws that controlled pretty much every activity of its citizens' lives. These laws were enacted by the Spartan King Lycurgus who is credited with having invented Sparta's unusual constitution.

Lycurgus' radical reinventing of Sparta probably occurred around the seventh century BCE. I say probably because even Lycurgus' biographer Plutarch can't make sense of the conflicting reports of when in history Lycurgus was king, giving himself the perfect get-out clause that I wish I'd thought of first. 'The history of these times is such a maze.'[8] I hear you, Plutarch, I hear you.

Lycurgus could have been knocking about with the poet Homer,[9] or before the first Olympic Games, or during the Bronze Age with the heroes of Homer's poetry, or he could have been two men called Lycurgus who lived at entirely different times and have been amalgamated into one dude. It's a big fat question mark. Which is odd, because despite not knowing when Lycurgus was knocking around, we do know a fair amount about what he did. What he did was restructure the entirety of Spartan society and as a result created an awful lot of laws.

It's odd that Sparta should feature so heavily in the culture of the USA because they couldn't be more diametrically opposed in ethos. America, as it likes to tell the rest of the world, is the land of the free and of freedom. Sparta was a totalitarian and authoritarian state where the government controlled every aspect of a Spartan's life. Freedom of choice and individualism were concepts utterly alien to the Spartans.

This control by the state over the life of their citizens began at birth. The exposure of infants, abhorrent as it is to us, was not uncommon in the ancient world. The first-century CE gynaecologist Soranus has a whole list of what to look for in a newborn baby in order to decide whether it was worth rearing and by rearing, I mean whether the baby should be welcomed as the newest member of your family or whether the baby would be taken away and left out on a street or hillside to die. Although there was always the slim possibility a childless couple might happen to be passing and take the child home with them. Or else a slave trader looking for free stock.

Greek mythology is awash with tales of the former, both Oedipus and Paris were exposed as babies, both were discovered by friendly shepherds who adopted them as their own child. Later they would both be reunited with their royal birth families in what you might imagine would be a happy ending but was instead, in both cases, an absolute catastrophe. Oedipus' 'happy' family reunion involved him inadvertently murdering his father and marrying his mother. Which is chicken feed to Paris, who shortly after being happily reunited with his Trojan birth parents and accepted into their palatial home, kidnapped/eloped with Helen of Troy and so brought about the destruction of Troy and the death of pretty much his entire family. Perhaps such catastrophic tales acted as a cautionary warning to every person who passed by a crying baby expelled from its family home because it was not considered worth rearing.

Soranus describes in some detail how to examine a newborn to determine whether it will be the latest addition to your family or not. You should check its joints and their movements, you should rate its cries as being sufficiently vigorous or not, ending with this chilling line: 'Conditions contrary to those mentioned, the infant not worth rearing is recognised.'[10]

Where Sparta differs in its attitudes to exposing infants is who got to make that decision. 'Offspring was not reared at the will of the father, but was taken by him to a place called Lesche, where the elders of the tribes officially examined the infant, and if it were well built and sturdy, they ordered the father to rear it.'[11] If the Spartan elders found the child less than impressive, they sent it to Mount Taygetus 'in the conviction that the life of that which nature had not well equipped at the beginning for health and strength, was of advantage either to itself or the state'.[12] The baby was then tossed into a chasm located at the foot of the mountain. No chance here of being picked up by a kindly shepherd or even a slave trader.

The crucial point here is that the decision to rear a child was taken away from the child's father, who in every other ancient society was the person who made that decision, as the head and ruler of family and who had, in some circumstances, power of life and death over the members of that family. Not in Sparta, in Sparta the state was the parent.

The chasm at the foot of Mount Taygetus, despite sounding like a destination straight out of *Lord of the Rings*, is an actual place situated in the Peloponnesian area of Greece. Archaeologists have been there, they have dug in the very chasm that Plutarch mentions and yes, they have found bodies, forty-six of them so far, dating back to the fifth and sixth centuries BCE. Only all of those bodies are of adults, not infants. Not a single body of an infant has been found.[13]

I have spent ten years writing about ancient history and many more years studying it, and do you know how rare it is to be able to comprehensively prove or disprove anything an ancient author says? It's as rare as winning the lottery two weeks running when you haven't bought a ticket. Writing about antiquity is to hedge your bets – yes, so and so author is probably making that tale up, but the hard evidence to prove that he is doesn't exist.[14] That we can say for definite that Plutarch is talking rubbish about the Spartans throwing their babies down mountains into a chasm beneath is extremely satisfying. I feel very satisfied. We needn't be too hard on Plutarch, he's writing several hundred years after Sparta's peak in the fifth century BCE, a time where young Spartan youths would re-enact the supposed customs of their forebears for tourists. This perhaps involved some form of staged re-enactment of the ceremony where the Spartan elders ruled that a new Spartan had been born.

Sparta was a closed society, strangers were not welcome there and Spartans themselves were not allowed to travel unless for war. 'It was not allowed them to go abroad, so that they should have nothing to do with foreign ways and undisciplined modes of living.'[15] From such circumstances details get exaggerated and invented. Most likely Sparta practised the exposure of infants as much as antiquity did, but they didn't do it from Mount Taygetus. Even if the power to decide whether to rear a child or not was given to the Spartan state, they certainly didn't exercise it to its fullest extent, disposing of every child considered less than perfect, because the Spartan king Agesilaus II, who ruled from 400 to 360 BCE, is widely credited with having been born lame in one leg. Maybe they made an exception for a son of a king or maybe it's another one of those Spartan myths, we'll hit several of them throughout this book.

We do have more contemporary sources for the height of Sparta's might than Plutarch, who is looking at a theme park version of Sparta, the equivalent of documenting medieval society using Disney films as your template. The reforms of Lycurgus are commented on by the likes of Plato and Xenophon who both lived during the time of Sparta's victory in the Peloponnesian Warand brief stance as the dominant city state in all of Greece.

Xenophon is a man to be envied, he was born in Athens probably around 431 BCE and died probably around 356 BCE, a period which coincided with that extraordinary explosion of brilliance that so affected sensitive poet types in the eighteenth century that they gushed out lines of verse and generally woe-ed about greatness they would never experience. Xenophon experienced the greatness of Classical Athens first hand, and his varied life reflected this. He was a successful military general of some talents, he was a friend and pupil of the philosopher Socrates and recorded many of his utterings for our benefit, he was a writer of history, of philosophy, a documenter of that extraordinary time in that extraordinary city.

Xenophon was present at the first stirrings of Western civilisation, stirrings that would inspire men for millennia. Only somewhat surprisingly, our man on the ground, our eyewitness to this pivotal moment in the history of the world we live in today, did not gush like the Romantic poets about the greatness around him (excluding Socrates, he gushes a lot about Socrates, it's pretty much a gushfest), instead he thought Sparta was much better. Sparta, whose contribution to our modern society is to give its name to a load of towns in the USA and be the subject of a truly dreadful film, *300*, which I'm still aggrieved at forking out money to go see.

'It occurred to me one day that Sparta, though among the most thinly populate of states was evidently the most powerful and celebrated city in Greece, and I fell to wondering how this could have happened. But when I consider the constitutions of the Spartans I wonder no longer,'[16] muses Xenophon, the inhabitant of a city that has recently introduced a political system that will be the aspiration for most of mankind, inspiring revolutionaries, political thinkers and poets.

Xenophon served as a mercenary soldier under Spartan commanders and was a friend of the Spartan king Agesilaus II.[17] The Spartans gave him a nice piece of land to live off as a reward for his service. Athens, his home nation, exiled him for the crime of having fought alongside the Spartans. His experience at the hands of Athens and Sparta no doubt colours his views. Sparta had been kind to him. Athens had not. So although Xenophon is our man on the ground in Sparta, let's just keep in mind that he may be putting a bit of a gleam on what he saw, whilst lugging around one big grudge against Athens. Disclaimer issued, let us hear out Xenophon on what is so great about Sparta.

Xenophon is particularly admiring of the Spartan educational system which he feels is far superior to the rest of Greece. In Sparta boys were taken away from their family at 7 years of age and enrolled into vigorous military training. Again, the state has taken on the role traditionally held by a parent, the state raises Spartan boys, not the child's parents, and the state's prime educational aim was to produce soldiers. This made the Spartan educational system very different to anything anywhere else in Greece. To say Spartan schooling was harsh is to describe Vlad the Impaler as misunderstood or Jack the Ripper as a bit naughty; it was brutal.

Athenian Xenophon fully approved of the brutal nature of the Spartan education system because he felt that other city states were far too indulgent to their children, pampering and spoiling them. How spoilt are these spoilt little brats? Well… 'Moreover, they soften the children's feet by giving them sandals and pamper their bodies with changes of clothing and it is customary to allow them as much food as they can eat!'[18]

Sparta did not spoil its children with luxuries like shoes and food. Spartan boys were forbidden to wear shoes to harden their feet, they were given only one type of garment to wear whatever the season to make them 'better prepared to face changes of heat and cold',[19] and were underfed so they would be used to hunger, be slimmer in figure and to 'make the boys more resourceful in getting supplies'.[20] By more resourceful he means stealing, Spartan boys were starved to desperation levels of hunger.

Although stealing was encouraged, being caught doing so was very much not. Plutarch recounts this horrific tale: 'the boys make such a serious matter of their stealing, that one of them, as they story goes, who was concealing a young fox he had stolen, suffered the animal to tear out his bowels with its teeth and claws and died rather than having his theft detected'.[21]

Xenophon is clear in his belief that this made the Spartans better soldiers than poncing about down the Athenian gym with your mates, distracted by all the gossip, philosophy and ball games going on all around you, and you can see why he might think that. What's a little discomfort whilst on campaign when you've never known anything different your entire life? Spartans from childhood were raised to be soldiers, there were no farmers or shepherds or accountants in ancient Sparta.[22] There were only soldiers, men who'd been brutalised since childhood into being perfect killing machines, happy to sacrifice themselves for the good of Sparta. An unstoppable, undefeated and damn right scary enemy to have. Or so the stories go.

The reality was a little different. The Spartans very successfully cultivated an image both in their own time and in ours that they were a perfect military force with strong notions of honour that have inspired generations of men from Xenophon all the way to Hitler, Elon Musk and all those teenage boys who went gleefully to repeat screenings of *300*. But it's an image that doesn't hold up to scrutiny.

Sparta was not an undefeated enemy of honourable heroes.[23] There are battles they did not win and less than honourable Spartan behaviour that appear repeatedly in our sources that we somehow overlook because we want to believe in the Spartan myth. Possibly because we are, like Xenophon, dissatisfied with the functioning of our own society and seeking a different way of living. Or else our own weaknesses have us gulping up stories about a land inhabited by men of courage and honour, the kind of men we wish we were.

Chapter 5
Greek Love

The previous chapters of this book covered the body beautiful, focusing in on the toned naked flesh of men coated in olive oil that glistened in the sun as they hung out with their fellow naked citizens in the gymnasium. Perhaps these adonises of antiquity would have a wrestle with each other, take part in a ball game, practise their discus-throwing skills, but before partaking in all these activities they would carefully tie their foreskins down, for reasons unknown.

There's been a question hanging in the air throughout the last few chapters on this male bodily perfection that so far has remained unaddressed. I know what you're thinking, because I'm thinking it too, anyone would. All these men doing manly things together in the nude, isn't it all a bit homoerotic? A bit, dare we say, gay? The answer is both yes, it is and no, it's not. Which will make perfect sense to you by the end of this chapter, I hope.

The work is called *Symposium*, and it was written by the philosopher Plato sometime around 385–370 BCE. The setting is the ancient Greek version of a dinner party which was known as a *symposium* (we will be looking at the *symposium* in more depth in the next chapter and explaining why it bears little resemblance to any dinner party you've ever been invited to or ever would want to be invited to), the guest list at this particular *symposium* includes a couple of people we've stumbled across before, the comic playwright Aristophanes and the philosopher Socrates, along with several other men who are not famous to us and so not worth naming at this point.

One of these guests at Plato's imaginary *symposium*, Eryximachus, has a suggestion about how they might entertain themselves that evening, and disappointingly it doesn't involve suspiciously under-dressed flute girls and a pot of honey. Nor does Eryximachus' suggestion involve getting smashed, because the same people, it appears, went to a much funner party the night before and did exactly that. 'I entirely agree, said Aristophanes, that we should, by all means, avoid hard drinking, for I was myself one of those who were yesterday drowned in drink.'[1]

This is what Eryximachus thinks will make it a fun evening for the very hungover guests. 'I mean to propose that each of us in turn, going from left to right, shall make a speech in honour of Love.'[2] Shudder. It's an icebreaker to send a chill into the soul of every British person forced to attend their work team-bonding away day. But this is ancient Athens and they love this sort of talking exercise, even with gruesome hangovers, in a way I find quite incomprehensible. I'm betting they were well up for charades too. Shudder.

Each of the guests then give their speech on love with thoughtful consideration. Phaedrus argues that love creates honour. 'I say that a lover who is detected in doing any dishonourable act, or submitting through cowardice when any dishonour is done to him by another, will be more pained at being detected by his beloved than at being seen by his father, or by his companions, or by anyone else.'[3] This sense of shame inspires men into noble acts and dispels cowardice, so argues Phaedrus. 'Love will make men dare to die for their beloved.'[4]

For Pausanias, love is more than bodily want, 'evil is the vulgar lover who loves the body rather than the soul.'[5] In Pausanias' speech the elder lover in a couple is responsible for educating the younger and guiding them through the world. 'This is that love which is the love of the heavenly goddess, and is heavenly, and of great price to individuals and cities, making the lover and the beloved alike eager in the work of their own improvement.'[6] All of which sounds a lot less fun than sharing a box of popcorn and having a bit of a snog on the back seat of the cinema. Pausanias' version of love, you sense, is going to come with homework and possibly an exam at the end to measure how much of your character has been improved.

These speeches go on for quite some time, which is impressive given they are speaking on the spot and all claim to be horribly hungover. Ancient Athenians are in a class of their own when it comes to wordiness, their best man speeches likely lasted for bum-aching hours. What is noticeable and unavoidable in the two speeches in praise of love I've mentioned so far is that the love they are largely describing is not between a man and a woman, but rather between men. Phaedrus' honourable lovers are men. 'And if there were only some way of contriving that a state or an army should be made up of lovers and their loves, they would be the very best governors of their own city, abstaining from all dishonour, and emulating one in honour; and when fighting at each other's side, although a mere handful, they would overcome the world.'[7]

Pausanias' younger partner being guided by the elder? Both male. 'Those who are inspired by this love turn to the male, and delight in him who is the more valiant and intelligent nature; anyone may recognise the pure enthusiasts in the very character of their attachments.'[8] Women do get a mention, a passing mention, but the bulk is on the superiority of same-sex partnerships as the purest form of love. It is from Plato, and particularly Pausanias' speech that heightens the intellectual as opposed to the bodily love for a person, that we get the phrase 'platonic love' from. Platonic love is not physical, it does not involve sex, rather it is the love of character, personality, the very essence and soul of a human being.

Aside from gifting posterity a word to describe a form of love we are familiar with today, Plato's *Symposium* also served as a kind of gay nirvana for men living through times that were very far from that. In E. M. Forster's posthumously published novel *Maurice*, the title character's university friend, Clive, makes a pass at him using Plato's work.

> 'I knew you read *Symposium* in the vac,' he said in a low voice.
> Maurice felt uneasy.
> 'Then you understand without me saying more.'
> 'How do you mean?'
> ... 'I love you.'[9]

Plato's *Symposium* and another of his works, *Phaedrus*, for the homosexual-leaning Clive, are a revelation. 'Never could he forget his emotion at first reading Phaedrus. He saw there his malady described exquisitely, calmly, as a passion which we can direct like any other towards good or bad.'[10]

You can see the appeal of Plato for both Clive and his creator E. M. Forster, who shared Clive's predilection; they were living in an era where homosexuality was illegal. Forster started writing Maurice in 1913, only eighteen years after the prosecution of Oscar Wilde for gross indecency for his relationships with men. The judge's opening lines to Wilde after the guilty verdict was announced give a stark picture of how homosexuality was viewed in this era.

> Oscar Wilde … the crime of which you have been convicted is so bad that one has to put stern restraint upon oneself to prevent oneself from describing, in language which I would rather not use, the sentiments which must rise in the breast of every man of honour who has heard the details.[11]

To the judge, Wilde was a man who had stepped across the line marked 'decent and honourable society' and dived headfirst into a pit of steaming manure from which he could never claw himself out. 'It is no use for me to address you. People who can do these things must be dead to all sense of shame, and one cannot hope to produce any effect upon them.'[12]

In such a climate it's no wonder that Clive and Forster found solace in Plato. 'For I know not any greater blessing to a young man who is beginning life than a virtuous lover or to the lover than a beloved youth.'[13] Here was what they felt, what the judge in Wilde's trial could barely describe for disgust, being talked about so matter-of-factly and openly, no shame involved.

In Aristophanes' speech later on in the *Symposium*, when he is talking about the two sexes, he throws in the line, 'by the mutual embraces of man and woman they might breed, and the race might continue; or if man came to man they might be satisfied, and rest, and go their ways to the business of life.'[14] Oscar Wilde's man-to-man satisfaction had led him to two years' hard labour in prison. In Plato's Greece it was something to be earnestly discussed at dinner parties and partaken in if one fancied it so. This was both shocking and revelatory.

So shocking and revelatory that the youth must be protected from exposure to it. Mr Cornwallis, Greek Literature Tutor to Maurice and Clive, instructs them to omit a passage relating to the 'Greek vice'. The Greek vice as depicted by Plato may have inspired and given hope to Clive and Maurice, but it was not homosexuality as we understand it today or as Clive and Maurice understand it to be, that of a mutually agreed partnership between two people of the same sex who happen to fall in love with one another. The Greek vice is a complicated topic that needs careful unpacking.

The ideal

> It is beautiful, it is fine, it is the noblest form of affection. There is nothing unnatural about it. It is intellectual, and it repeatedly exists between an elder and a younger man, when the elder man has intellect, and the younger man has all the joy, hope and glamour of life before him. That it should be so the world does not understand. The world mocks at it and sometimes puts one in the pillory for it.[15]

So said Oscar Wilde about this so-called Greek vice, which going forward I shall now refer to as Greek love, and it really gets to the heart of what Wilde also dubs 'the love that dare not speak its name' was all about.

In ancient Greece it was less the love that dare not speak its name and more the love we are going to spend hours debating during a dinner party, write lots of poetry about and splash all over our crockery. There is a lot of evidence for the existence of relationships between men in ancient Greece, but as with all source material we need to be quite cautious about what we are seeing and being told and crucially who is doing the telling.

What Oscar Wilde and Plato's party guests describe is a very particular type of relationship between men with a very particular set of societal rules and norms structured around it. These were relationships that were of interest to the *polis* and served as part of a young man's transition and initiation into manhood and public life. The case we are looking at below is based on Athenian rituals and social norms, other parts of Greece had their own customs as we shall see later.

The first rule was that in these relationships there would be a considerable age difference; the younger man was known as an *eromenos* and the older man an *erastes*. The job of the *erastes* was to act as a mentor to the *eronemos* and to pass onto him the skill set needed to become a fully functioning paid-up member of the *polis*. The role of the *erastes* was a crucial one therefore, one of moulding potential new citizens and ensuring they didn't go off the rails as young men sometimes do when they hit peak testosterone.

As Pausanias says in the Symposium, the *eromenos* will be improved in wisdom and virtue, a decent citizen of the *polis* in other words. The *erastes* is a mentor, a positive male role model for the young man. However, before he could mentor all the fun out of youth the *erastes* had to first find himself that perfect mouldable splodge of young playdoh to work with. The place to find your *eromenos* was the same place you found everything else of value in ancient Greece, the gymnasium!

'I am not ashamed that I am a pest in the gymnasium and have been a lover to so many boys,'[16] says Aeschines, making the whole bagging a mentee thing sound easy. We know that not every would-be *erastes* was blessed with Aeschines' easy swagger and pick-up abilities, we know that there was considerable competition between men for the best mouldable *eromenos* material, we even know the names of some of the most sought-after mentees. In Athens in 520 BCE, the most popular boy at the gym was Leagros, we know this because his name is plastered all over crockery, apparently Leagros is beautiful. Beautiful enough to keep potters busy all over Athens; perhaps Leagros himself was the recipient of some of these vases, a gift to win him over. To win Leagros you needed a lot of gifts and charm and honeyed words.

The famously beautiful Alcibiades, of whom his biographer Plutarch says, 'As regards the beauty of Alcibiades, it is perhaps unnecessary to say aught, except that it flowered out with each successive season of his bodily growth, and made him, alike in boyhood, youth and manhood, lovely and pleasant,'[17] was another favoured youth of the season. 'Many men of high birth clustered about him and paid him attention.'[18] Although Alcibiades, being the contrary creature he was – he swapped sides during the Peloponnesian War twice – settles his attentions on an *erastes* who has no interest in him, the philosopher Socrates.

Now studies in our own time have repeatedly shown the positive benefits of a male role model on young men[19] with accompanying newspaper headlines worrying about the lack of male teachers at primary-level schooling and elsewhere in society. Alcibiades certainly saw the benefits to himself, and his character, particularly to be gained from his relationship with Socrates. 'And he came to think that the work of Socrates was really a kind of provision of the gods for the care and salvation of youth,'[20] chiefly because Socrates 'sought to expose the weakness of his soul and rebuke his vain and foolish pride'. The kind of vanity and pride that come with being so absolutely drop-dead gorgeous that Plutarch, writing 600 years later, feels 'as regards the beauty of Alcibiades, it is perhaps unnecessary to say aught' because everybody is still aware of that he was bloody phwoarness of the flesh.

That the *eromenos* was apparently the chief beneficiary of this arrangement, as Alcibiades was, the one who received all the wisdom and knowledge of the *erastes*, who gained the leg-up in society from a powerful well-connected man, throws up two questions: first, why did the *erastes* court the *eromenos* and not the other way round? And secondly if the *eromenos* receives all the wisdom and knowledge of the *erastes*, how does the *erastes* benefit? What's in it for him?

We could take the altruistic route and say that the *erastes* gains by successfully moulding his *eromenos* for public life, watching his pupil grow into a full-fledged member of the *polis* and taking pride in his accomplishments, knowing that he was behind that success. But more importantly, everyone else knowing that too. Duty, pride and smugness are a powerful triad of motivations. Oscar Wilde, as we saw at the opening of this chapter, saw the benefits for the older partner being an enjoyment of youth: 'the younger man has all the joy, hope and glamour of life before him.' In Phaedra's speech in the *Symposium* the *eromenos* brings out the finer qualities of his mentor in the shape of physical courage, an attribute so prized in ancient Greece.

If this is sounding a bit too perfect, a bit too noble, a bit too altruistic, a bit too unbelievable that an adult Greek male would selflessly give up hours of workout time/getting pissed with his mates to endlessly court and then coach a handsome young stranger in how to be a good citizen for absolutely no recompense, you are entirely right. On the not entirely altruistic side, we have seen there was lustre to be gained by attracting the most beautiful youth to your mentoring side, the *erastes* could improve his reputation and his standing within the polis. But there was more in it for the *erastes* than a bit of showing off to his chums, because Greek love was not the platonic, hands-off, intellectual meeting of mind and souls its most fervent admirers have gushed over across the centuries.

Now is the time to flick back to our basics on Greek society, and more particularly those multitude of words the Greeks employed for love, because it's going to help make a little more sense of Greek love. The word you find employed most readily for this relationship between *eromenos* and *erastes* is not agape, which was the word Jesus Christ used for the disciples he was schooling in doctrine and a new way of living, it was *eros*. Agape was truly platonic love, *eros* could involve a passionate physical love. There was sex involved in Greek love.

The crack in the vase

It's odd that it is Plato who should lend his name to a phrase describing a non-sexual relationship, because in the *Symposium*, although much is made of the virtuous duty of the *erastes*, it is clear there is a payoff for his virtuous acts. 'And these two customs, one the love of youth, and the other the practice of philosophy and virtue in general, ought to meet in one, and then the beloved may honourably indulge the lover.'[21]

'Indulge' is a very vague word. Alternative translations of the *Symposium* use the phrase 'grant favours'. Either way, the *eromenos* is giving something to his *erastes* by way of payment for all that character building and wisdom he has received. 'He who gives himself to a lover because he is a good man, and in the hope that he will be improved by his company, shows himself to be virtuous.'[22]

This is not platonic love. This is not the story of an older man altruistically mentoring a youth, it's a deal with obligations on both sides. The *erastes* provides a service for which the *eromenos* is expected to honour by 'indulging' and 'favour granting'. I think we can all guess what those favours granted might be.

In one of Plato's other works, *Phaedrus*, physical relations between men are referred to constantly. 'What is more, most lovers develop a desire for the body first, before they have come to know your character or your other personal qualities, so that it is not clear whether they will still want to be friends with you once the passion has abated.'[23]

In *Phaedrus*, the discussion centres around the speech of a certain Lysias, who argues that it is better to have sexual relations with someone who does not love you because love clouds the judgement of men. 'In the case of those who are not lovers but were friends with one another before all this took place, the friendship is not likely to be diminished by any of their pleasant experiences, but these are likely to be left as memorials for what is about to unfold.'[24]

These 'pleasant experiences' are not defined any more graphically than that. For all the use of the word love and lovers and all the talk around courting, securing beauty and the benefits of love, there is a noticeable lack of words given to the physical act of love. I guess this censorship of words is to be expected, given one of our chief sources for relations between men is a philosopher, a man who expresses thoughts and ideas rather than actions. Plato is hardly going to write a sex guide. He should have. It would have saved a great deal of debate amongst academics across the centuries.

We do, however, have other sources at our disposal to try and decipher what sex between an *eromenos* and *erastes* might have involved, such as the wealth of pottery depicting everyday life that has survived. As noted in a previous chapter, Greek men are depicted doing a lot of activities naked together, which can make interpreting the multitude of scenes we see depicted on Greek vases open to misunderstanding, unsurprisingly so. This is a culture dating back over 2,000 years and there's not a lot of writing on vases to aid us in our interpretations, no handy arrow pointing at two naked men with the caption 'wrestlers' that clear the matter up unequivocally for us. Therefore, we must be cautious in making sweeping conclusions on what we see or what we don't see depicted on Greek vases. There's an additional complication in remembering that these vases had a purchaser and a creator who needed to make a living by producing vases that would sell.

It is important to recognise that these vases were originally produced for a mass market of ordinary Greeks, a fact that can be easily overlooked given their current display in our most prestigious museums. Their august settings make us view them differently in the twenty-first century, to us they are art and a window into another culture. Neither of which is how they were viewed back in ancient Greece; they were practical everyday objects that people brought for a practical purpose.

Imagine future historians trying to understand twenty-first-century society using only the shards of surviving coffee mugs discovered in the remnants of gift shops across the land. What could they possibly conclude other than twenty-first-century Britain was a nation to whom the natural world of pretty flowers was paramount, homage regularly paid to ancient structures and the existence of a mysterious cult called the National Trust that had infiltrated nearly all sectors of society? It doesn't offer up a thorough picture of modern Britain, does it? Nor do Greek vases. Probably the only definitive statement we can make about the scenes depicted on Greek vases is that, like gift shop mugs, they appealed to the masses.

Having issued the necessary disclaimer, let us now look at depictions of Greek love on Greek vases. First things first, what you won't find are any depictions of anal sex between older and younger men, or between adult male citizens at all.[25] You won't on British gift shop mugs either, in case you were wondering, although I'm not entirely ruling it out. One place where you do find anal sex represented on Greek pottery is between satyrs.

Satyrs are mythical creatures who drew the short straw for dignity in the lexicon of half-human/half-animals that proliferate in Greek mythology. They are no sleek centaur with a practical horse bottom half that ups their speediness, nor a terrifying gorgon like Medusa and her snazzy snake hair-do, but rather unattractive-looking human men with the hairy legs of some kind of an animal, a tail that might be from a horse or even a donkey, pointed ears to make Mr Spock proud and a permanent erection which is on full display since satyrs, like ancient Greek men, have an aversion to clothing.

Satyrs are comic figures, always up to mischief and generally partaking in activities that should be labelled 'things that'll land you in the Accident and Emergency Department later'. These include balancing glassware on their erections, attempting to have sex with pretty much anything, including wine skins, deer, other animals and often each other. Very unwisely, satyrs also try their luck with nymphs. I say unwisely since nymphs are often portrayed armed with a thyros (a staff topped with a pinecone, as was sacred to the god of wine and fun, Dionysius, and his followers) which they are clearly going to use to beat the crap out of any horny satyr, quite possibly in his enlarged lap area. Satyrs serve as a warning as not what to do and how not to behave. Images 28 and 29, depicting alternate sides of the same cup, perfectly encapsulate the satyr's lot in life; on one side the satyr chases after a nymph, intent on having her, on the alternate side he is being chased away by the victim of his lust. That satyrs have large, ungainly penises is sign enough of their barbarism and lack of civilisation.

Aside from satyrs, we find anal sex depicted between men and prostitutes, again relations that although a feature of Greek society are not presented as an ideal. But also between men and women who are not prostitutes, which maybe says something about the lingering influence of Greek love upon the sexual appetites of Greek men and the passive role women were expected to adhere to in Greek society. Or alternatively the missionary position gave less scope for the vase painter to depict boobs, bums and cocks as clearly as his clientele demanded. It's open to debate, which I would, but I have a set word count and too many things to say on this subject. Let us move on.

So that's where we do find depictions of anal sex. Where we don't find it depicted, interestingly enough, is in representations of Greek love. Having stated just a few lines earlier the dangers of using vases and other surviving pottery to make sweeping statements of definitive fact about ancient Greek culture, I will refrain from making any. I will, however, raise my eyebrows and give you a look that strongly suggests you take note of this because it might be important later.

What we do find on a certain subsection of Greek pottery is depictions of the *eromenos* and *erastes* together. We can decipher which is which because the *erastes* is depicted with a full bushy beard of the type ancient Greek men were hugely fond of, and the *eromenos* is clean-shaven and considerably smaller in stature. In these scenes the *eromenos* is also usually naked, the *erastes* sometimes, sometimes not. How do we know that this is Greek love in action and not an older man simply having a chat with a young fellow at the gym? Because the *erastes* has his hand on the *eromenos*' genitals and he has an erection. You won't find any depiction of an *eromenos* sexually aroused because he is the passive party in the relationship, the passive part is important, crucially so, as again we'll see a bit later on in this chapter. The *eromenos* has been the courted in this relationship, the recipient of gifts and compliments: he is the passive, and indeed flaccid recipient of physical love. You'll remember in our chapter on the language of love that *eros* was not mutual love and nowhere is this clearer than in the dealings between an *erastes* and his *eromenos*. The *eromenos* is the recipient of *eros* from his *erastes*, he is not expected to feel it and certainly not to show it himself.

The much-courted, handsome Alcibiades' choice of Socrates as his *erastes* is described as, 'giving ear to the words of a lover who was in the chase for no unmanly pleasures, and begged no kisses and embraces, but sought to expose the weakness of his soul and rebuke his vain and foolish pride'.[26]

Making it clear that others of his suitors were very much in it for the kisses and embraces.

This physical love, as far as we can make out in the case of Athens, did not involve penetrative anal sex, nor oral sex. Instead, what occurred between them was intercrural sex, where the *erastes* positioned his penis between the thighs of the *eromenos* and thrust away until ejaculation. Intercrural sex we do find depicted on Greek vases and other pottery.

That nothing more physical is found depicted could point two directions, it could be because this was as physical as relations got in Greek love, or it could be that it got a lot more physical but everyone wanted to pretend that it didn't. One reason for this silence might be to protect the future reputation of the *eromenos* who had been mentored the hell into a prominent role in the life of the *polis*, a role he was unlikely to be considered for had it been known he had been anally penetrated by another man; such an act cast him as passive as a woman and thus of dubious character.

The *erastes* might find himself the butt of jokes for being unsuccessful in courting the popular *eromenos* of the season, but it was the latter that was in most danger. The *eromenos* had to balance offering enough to his mentor to ensure his support in his public career, but not so much as to reveal himself to be of a wanton character. He had to be both virtuous and put out, which is quite some challenge.

Where the line lay between acceptable physical relations and unacceptable physical relations is the subject of a court case brought by Aeschines against a man named Timarchus in 345 BCE. There were political reasons why Aeschines had put together a case against Timarchus, it was pure malice/revenge for a case brought against him for misconduct whilst he'd been an ambassador to Philip II of Macedon. Aeschines' charges against Timarchus are that he had exhibited behaviour of such immorality that it disqualified him from being a member of the Athenian Assembly. You're now all gagging to know what Timarchus had been up to, aren't you? Or rather what Aeschines claimed he'd been up to.

Aeschines handily quotes the law that Timarchus has allegedly breached:

> If any Athenian shall have prostituted his person, he shall not be permitted to become one of the nine archons, nor to discharge the office of priest, nor

> to act as an advocate for the state, nor shall he hold any office whatsoever, at home or abroad, whether filled by lot or by election; he shall not be sent as a herald; he shall not take part in debate, nor be present at public sacrifices; when the citizens are wearing garlands, he shall wear none; and he shall not enter within the limits of the place that has been purified for the assembling of the people. If any man who has been convicted of prostitution act contrary to these prohibitions, he shall be put to death.[27]

Timarchus was facing prosecution for selling bodily favours, a crime considered so serious that it excluded him from participating in civic society and all that involved, which is carefully listed to ensure anyone convicted knows where they are not wanted. Timarchus was facing expulsion from public life entirely, which in status-conscious Athens is a pretty harsh punishment. You can tell how harsh it is because the convicted must be threatened with execution to prevent them from accidentally wandering into the assembly and casting a vote or stumbling across a public sacrifice and absentmindedly donning a garland.

There is a strange contradiction here: it is illegal in Athens to grant sexual favours in exchange for something of value, whilst the societal norm in Athens is for younger men to grant sexual favours to older men in exchange for mentoring, which is portrayed in our sources as being of great value. That's a line so thin as to be invisible to the naked eye, especially when you factor in the gift lavishing during the courting phase of Greek love. This narrow line between the virtue of Greek love and the vice of male prostitution is something that Aeschines seeks to distinguish in his prosecution speech. 'I will recite to you the names of older and well-known men, and of youths and boys, some of whom have had many lovers because of their beauty, and some of whom, still in their prime, have lovers today, but not one of whom ever came under the same accusations as Timarchus.'[28]

The specific instance cited against Timarchus is that he lived with a series of men, firstly with a man named Misgolas and then others afterwards, because he was paid to do so. That Aeschines is lacking actual evidence of this is peppered throughout his speech.

> My fellow citizens, I call upon you to make your decision in this case in the same manner. In the first place, let nothing be more credible in your eyes than

> your own knowledge and conviction regarding this man Timarchus. In the second place, look at the case in the light, not of the present moment, but of the time that is past. For the words spoken before today about Timarchus and his practices were spoken because they were true; but what will be said today will be spoken because of the trial, and with intent to deceive you. Give, therefore, the verdict that is demanded by the longer time, and the truth, and your own knowledge.[29]

So basically, telling the jury to make free with their own preconceptions and prejudices against the defendant and to totally ignore any evidence brought up in the trial he is the prosecutor of, because that'll all be lies. Never has the phrase the court of public opinion been truer, Timarchus is facing trial by gossip, gossip that Aeschines doesn't even helpfully define for the jury to aid their deliberations. 'For all the things that this man here was unashamed to do in deed. I would sooner die than describe in plain words in your presence.'[30] Which creates a neat blank space in the minds of the jury members who hadn't heard the gossip about Timarchus to mentally fill using their imagination.

Instructing the jury to convict the defendant based on what they have heard about him in conversations at the gym or in agora or at a *symposium* and then making vague references himself to Timarchus' behaviour is the only tactic Aeschines has open to him. We can deduce this because he doesn't present any evidence that Timarchus prostituted himself to the jury. He offers up a lot of hearsay, gossip and a whole heap of suggestion, which I like to imagine he delivered whilst raising one eyebrow. When he brings in Misgolas – one of the men that he alleges Timarchus sold his body to – to testify, at no point does Misgolas make any reference to payment changing hands for sexual favours. 'Misgolas, son of Nicias, of Piraeus, testifies. Timarchus, who once used to stay at the house of Euthydicis the physician, became intimate with me, and I hold him today in the same esteem as in all my past acquaintance with him.'[31]

Astonishingly, despite not having a case, Aeschines wins and Timarchus is banned from partaking in civic life and shamed before his peers forever more.

There are a number of lessons to be learnt from this trial: firstly, never piss off Aeschines, because whatever you dish out to him he's going to dish it straight back at you, with a massive ladle. Secondly, the burden of proof in Greek trials was considerably less stringent than today, with gossip being treated as if it has the substance of a matching DNA sample. And thirdly, your time as the *eromenos* to an *erastes* could be used against you at a later date should you have nudged even slightly to the left of the wafer-thin line that divided granting sexual favours for knowledge dispensed from a gift-bearing lover and the crime of prostitution.

What is a youth?

Having tackled one elephant in the room, the sex element, let us tackle that other trunked beast taking up space on the sofa: in the case of the *eromenos*, what do we mean by youth? Just how old are these youths being courted for possible sex by fully bearded adult men?

Pausanias' speech in the *Symposium* spells it out for us. 'For they love not boys, but intelligent beings whose reason is beginning to be developed, much about the time at which their beards begin to grow.'[32] Boys enter puberty at around 12 years of age, facial hair is one of the later of the changes a boy experiences, occurring around the age of 14–16 years of age. By our laws, the *eromenos* would be classed a child, unable to give consent.

This is a knotty, difficult subject, particularly at this point in the twenty-first century when many of our institutions, the Catholic church, the scouts, boarding schools and sports teams, have been exposed as having endemic levels of child sexual abuse. The word 'grooming' has entered our language to describe the manipulative acts of an adult to entice a child into sexual relations. A lot of what we have discussed in this chapter sounds like grooming to our twenty-first-century ears, and a lot of what we are going to hear sounds like the justification of that grooming. For example, this introduction to a chapter on homosexuality in ancient Greece: 'We have to clarify from the start that pederasty did not have a homosexual character and therefore should not be confused with paedophilia, the sexual abuse of children. The word pederasty denotes the spiritual affection and admiration for a boy, and in ancient Greece was not used obscenely.'[33]

Expressing 'spiritual affection and admiration for a boy' is a deeply suspect and troubling sentence for the modern reader, one that we struggle to not think of as sexual. The ideals of Greek love we touched on earlier in this chapter have found expression in our society, and not in a good way.

NAMBLA – the North American Man/Boy Love Association – buys into the rhetoric of the pure nature of Greek love. 'Man/boy relationships are based on mutual respect and affection, and strongly desired by both partners. Such relationships do not harm anyone, and often entail many benefits for both man and boy. Boy lovers and boys alike respond to the needs of those they love – needs for affection, understanding, and freedom.'[34]

It should be noted that on the same website that NAMBLA professes that man/boy relationships harm nobody, it also boasts that it is 'is the only organization that specifically supports incarcerated individuals who identify as boy lovers'. NAMBLA campaigns against the age of consent, declaring, 'We believe sexual feelings are a positive life force. We support the rights of youth as well as adults to choose the partners with whom they wish to share and enjoy their bodies.' Of course they do.

The 1970s in the UK saw the rise of the Paedophile Information Exchange which had similar aims to NAMBLA. It too campaigned for abolishing the age of consent and used language around allowing children to be sexual beings. It seems incredible from our vantage point that a pressure group that used the word paedophile in its name should ever have been allowed to operate, let alone gain traction, but it did. The Paedophile Information Exchange gave every Member of the British Parliament a copy of its booklet, 'Paedophilia; Some Questions and Answers'. Which is the perfect title for the opposite of a page turner of a book, it's a straight into the bin unread book, I'm not even curious as to what questions they could have possibly come up with that they imagined the British public had about paedophiles beyond: what is wrong with you?

The Paedophile Information Exchange produced a regular newsletter for its members which sought to justify the aims of the organisation, of children it said: 'They are often interested in adults' bodies and, from the age of about nine or ten, in adult's sex lives. They are quite capable of indulging in sex games with willing adults, and even of provoking or initiating them.'[35] Astonishingly it argued, 'there is no evidence that sexual contacts with adults do any damage, psychological or moral, to the children any more than the "rude games" that many of them play. There is considerable evidence that parental distress and police intervention do cause a great deal of harm.'

All the glossy language, the intellectual justifications and the claims of acting only in the best interests of children wasn't distracting enough to hide the true aim of the Paedophile Information Exchange – to facilitate sex with children for the personal sexual gratification of their members. Despite repeated tabloid front-page exposes on the group, its demise came about in a large part to the endeavours of Scottish headmaster Charles Oxley. Oxley joined the Paedophile Information Exchange with a singular mission, 'to bring these evil men to justice'. The dossier he handed to Scotland Yard in 1983 detailing what he had discovered about the group's activities sped up its death. The Paedophile Information Exchange disbanded in 1984.

A decade before the founding of the Paedophile Information Exchange, American preacher Daivd Berg founded his own cult known as the Children of God. Berg took the 1960s ethos of free love far beyond societal boundaries of acceptability. Members of the Children of God were taught that God was love and expressing that love between each other physically was to praise God. Part of its doctrine was, 'God loves sex because sex is love, and Satan hates sex because sex is beautiful.' Children of God leader, David Berg himself, declared that 'love has no age limit'. Escapees and survivors of the cult have provided plenty of horrifying material on how Berg's notions of free love for all had led to wide-scale child abuse within its walls.

Paedophile and paedophilia are words that evoke strong feelings of repulsion and disgust in the twenty-first century, which is why in more recent years we have seen the phrase 'minor attracted people' creeping into use under the banner of respecting the individual's sexual orientation. Critics of the term rightly point out this rebranding has the effect of sanitising and de-stigmatising child abusers, offering them up a readily available justification and excuse for their actions. It's not my fault, it's who I am – a line that appears frequently in the members' letters that the Paedophile Information Exchange published back in the 1970s and early 1980s.

There have always been paedophiles, and there have always been those set on justifying and excusing such behaviour. Which takes us back to ancient Athens and whether the ideals expressed of Greek love are similar to the ideals expressed by NAMBA, the Paedophile Information Exchange and the Children of God, simply an excuse, a smokescreen for adults to indulge their basest desires.

The reality

First things first, the era we are examining here is separated from our own by thousands of years, and it's a culture that despite its gifts to our civilisation (which we looked at in our first chapter) has a very different ethos to our own times. It does not share the bedrock of our society, Christianity, nor does it hold with our own romanticism and extension of childhood. The average age of a first-time bride in the UK in 2023 was 30, in ancient Greece girls were married at around 14 to husbands decades older than them. The age difference between the male couples involved in Greek love does not seem so shocking in the context of their times.

Despite the chasm between our two cultures, the ancient Greeks themselves recognised that Greek love was not necessarily the moral and pure mentorship it was portrayed as. Remember Oscar Wilde's words at his trial on the love that dare not speak its name? 'It is beautiful, it is fine, it is the noblest form of affection.' Wilde's expression of Greek love extended beyond his supposed great love Lord Alfred Douglas, it was expressed many times over in the gay underground world of Victorian London with poor, working-class young men who took the coins that Wilde handed to them after he'd engaged them in sexual activities.

As well as handing over cash for sex, Wilde plied these youths with alcohol to make them more amenable to his affections and then bought them presents. These gifts included shirts, handkerchiefs, a silver watch and chain, a silver cigarette case, a gold ring. His wealth was dazzling to these young men, as one Charles Parker testified during Wilde's trial. 'I said that if any old gentleman with money took a fancy to me, I was agreeable. I was agreeable. I was terribly hard up.'[36] Terribly hard up in Victorian London was to be utterly destitute and starving to the point at which you will do anything for money, anything just to survive.

For Edward Shelley, who worked at Wilde's publishers, it was not Wilde's money but rather his fame and influence that was used to coerce him into a hotel room with the writer. 'At first I thought that Mr. Wilde was a kind of philanthropist, fond of youth and eager to be of assistance to young men, of any promise.' Shelley was soon disabused of the notion that the attentions Wilde was paying to him were the altruist acts of a mentor.

Wilde doesn't seem so noble, so persecuted now, does he? He comes across as a predator dressed up in the guise of a benefactor, and the judge's denouncement and disgust at Wilde is rendered more understandable. Not to say that Victorian Britain wasn't a terrible place to be a homosexual, it most certainly was, but Oscar Wilde's reputation was savaged by his own sexual behaviour rather than purely by his sexuality (although obviously that played a part).

Just as Oscar Wilde's version of Greek love did not match up to his words, so it was the case in ancient Athens where there was also sleaziness going on. The law in Athens makes distinctions at age 18, with over-18s being liable for their own transgressions of the law and the father or guardian of the under-18s having to foot the bill for any fines. Under-18s were accompanied around the city by their *paidagogos*, a slave dedicated to their care.

There are some interesting laws that hint at the under-18s needing the protection of that *paidagogos*. 'The teachers of boys shall open their schoolrooms before sunrise and shall close them at sunset. And it shall not be permitted for anyone older than the boys to enter while the boys are inside, unless he be the teacher or a brother or a son in law.'[37] Which could be read as the ancient Athenians being extremely keen on their sons not having unnecessary interruptions to their school, at least until you get to the penalty for stepping into a school during class time. 'And if anyone should enter in contravention of these prohibitions he shall be punishable by death.'[38]

Another punishable offence was levelled at the gym owner who allowed any man of maturity to enter his gymnasium whilst those under 18 were exercising. The owner flouting this law was 'subject to the law that applies to the seduction of free born youth'.[39] Added to this was the crime of hubris committed against a free child which could result in your execution on the same day the accusation was raised against you. This was swift and brutal justice for an offence, hubris, which we don't fully understand; however, from the context in which we find it used, scholars have deduced it most likely referred to both physical and sexual assaults.

Alongside these laws there were others regarding prostitution and the potential of prostitution: 'the law says explicitly that if a father, brother, uncle, guardian or anyone at all who is responsible for a boy hires him out as a prostitute it does not allow a charge to be laid against the boy himself.'[40]

The picture being painted here is of a society well aware that its youth were at risk from sexual exploitation and sought to protect them from this threat. It's time to reflect upon those vase images of the older bearded man fondling the genitals of the clean-shaven younger man again; might they be less a depiction of Greek cultural norms and a visual warning of the danger from those creepy men who hang round the gym a young man might face?

How do we square this with all that we've covered in this chapter on the *erastes* and his *eromenos* as featured in Plato? James Davidson, in his doorstop of a book, *The Greeks and Greek Love*, has the perfect solution to square that circle: in ancient Greece, boys reached puberty at an older age than today with facial hair growth occurring at around age 18.[41] This is an enormously satisfying solution because it makes sense of all those Athenian laws that specifically apply to the protection of the under-18s from unwanted or forced sexual encounters. In one fell swoop, Davidson's suggestion frees the ancient Athenians from the accusation of socially normalised paedophilia.

However, studies of palaeolithic and medieval skeletons have shown that the onset of puberty in these eras is largely the same as in our own.[42] Which leaves us where? Perhaps with the conclusion that platonic love/Greek love, that love between two males with a heavy load of character improving and virtue endowing, was not as acceptable and as accepted by society as many Greek writers would have us believe. That there was a fear that such practices could be dangerous and damaging for a would-be *eromenos*.

With all this conflicting evidence, what conclusions can we safely make? Very few, I would say, with complete confidence. In Athens, the practice of Greek love was limited to a very small slice of society, the elite, this is very clear from our sources. The most beautiful boy of the year or men known for their youthful attractiveness are not the sons of carpenters or casual labourers, that is for sure. Then there is this law which hammers the message home on who was allowed to participate in Greek love. 'He also wrote a law forbidding a slave to practise gymnastics or have a boy lover, thus putting the matter in the category of honour and dignified practices, and in a way inciting the worthy to that which he forbade the unworthy.'[43]

Within this elite community, Greek love was controlled by societal conventions on how it should proceed, with strict laws hovering above ready to pounce on those who stood outside these controls. Although we have no evidence that any *erastes* was ever brought to prosecution for such transgressions.

Chapter 6

Greek Love Outside of Athens

We have so far looked at how Greek love and homosexuality were practised in Athens because that is where the majority of our sources come from. However, Greek love pertaining to a mentoring relationship between an adult male and a youth existed in other parts of Greece too but in slightly different forms.

Sparta

Although Spartan ideals and ideology are about as far removed from those of Athens as possible, nonetheless a very similar notion of Athenian Greek love was to be found in Sparta, introduced by the legendary (and likely fictious) lawmaker Lycurgus. 'If, someone being himself an honest man admired a boy's soul and tried to make of him an ideal friend without reapproach and tried to associate with him, he approved and believed in the excellence of this kind of training.'[1] So far, so Athenian-style personal ad: older bearded and wise man seeks attractive youth to inspire into being a better person. GSOH and ability to listen essential. However, according to Xenophon, the Spartan model of Greek love deviated from the Athenian model. 'If it was clear that the attraction lay in the outward beauty, he banned it as an abomination.'[2] To underline that this is a true thing and not merely the sort of wishful thinking Xenophon knows is present elsewhere in Grece, including his home city of Athens, he adds that Lycurgus 'caused lovers to abstain from boys no less than parents abstain from sexual intercourse with their children and brothers and sisters with each other'.[3] Which seemingly leaves in no doubt how strongly the Spartans felt about sexual relations between men and youths, it was considered as taboo as incest! You can probably sense I'm about to drop in a 'but' or a 'however' and you'd be correct in sensing that, here it comes…

However, there are certain elements of Spartan society that put into doubt Xenophon's bold statement. Even with the best will in the world, the Spartan model is ripe for abuse, as Roman statesmen Cicero, looking back from the first century BCE, comments: 'the Spartans themselves, who give every freedom to love relations with young men except that of actual defilement, protect only by a very thin wall this one exception, for, providing only that cloaks be interposed, they allow embraces and the sharing of the bed.'[4] I don't think I'm alone in sensing Cicero's scepticism that a cloak was any sort of deterrent or barrier to more intimate mentoring.

Heck, even Xenophon recognises some people will be sceptical that Spartan relations between men and boys were entirely chaste and proper. 'I am not surprised, however, that people refuse to believe this. For in many states the laws are not opposed to the indulgence of these appetites.'[5] Which suggests to me that Xenophon has held court at some *symposium* with his tales of Spartan sexual restraint and been ever so slightly hurt by the loud guffaws at his naivety.

Another one of Lycurgus' laws 'gave every father authority over other men's children as well as his own'.[6] This extended to physical punishment: 'if a boy tells his own father when he has been whipped by another father, it is a disgrace if the parent does not give his son another whipping.'[7] Alongside this was the position of Warden who was given the authority to 'gather boys together to take charge of them and to punish them severely in case of misconduct'.[8] If the Warden should happen to be away, his powers and authority were handed over to any other citizen who fancied a go at instigating proper conduct in Spartan boys. Effectively every adult male in Sparta had complete power to inflict whatever he liked over any boy he so wished, as Xenophon himself admits: 'At Sparta the boys are never without a ruler.'[9] Which is a safeguarding nightmare if ever I heard one.

Then there's the Spartan wedding ceremony which contains this odd element. 'The bride's-maid, so called, took her in charge, cut her hair off close to the head, put a man's cloak and sandals on her, and laid her down on a pallet, on the floor, alone, in the dark.'[10] The groom enters, takes her virginity and then after 'spending a short time with his bride, he went away composedly to his usual quarters, there to sleep with the other young men'.[11]

Paul Cartledge, the premier expert on ancient Sparta, ties this peculiar ritual to the Spartan desire to produce a strong race of masculine sons. Or alternatively, the likes of Xenophon's sceptical *symposium* guests (and you and I, I'm guessing) suspect that Spartan brides were dressed up as boys as a kindness, to ease the grooms into heterosexual relations which they were unfamiliar with. Spartan purists today, like Xenophon before them, can claim with some justification that Spartan boys were in exclusively male company from the age of 7, being moulded into perfect killing machines, and that was why. Whichever way you look at it, dressing a bride up as a boy specifically for the consummation of the marriage is weird, and hints at something untoward bubbling beneath the surface of Sparta's supposed moral purity.

The peculiarity of sexual relations between Spartan husbands and wives did not limit itself to the wedding night, it continued into their marriage (as we shall explore in a later chapter). For now, on the existence of same-sex relationships/Greek love in Sparta, firm conclusions cannot be made, but come on! This is a society where boys spend their peak testosterone years sharing quarters and the company of their fellow hormoned-up teenage boys, whilst being under the watch of adult male Spartans who happen to possess full authority over them and have been encouraged by the great Lycurgus from beyond the grave to admire the souls of such boys and initiate a 'friendship'… It's open to suspicion. I'm suspicious.

Crete

If you thought the Spartan wedding ceremony was, let us say, a bit odd then hold onto your cup of coffee lest it fly out your hands and ruin a perfectly nice sofa, because things are about to head in an even weirder direction on the island of Crete. Ancient Crete (we are talking post-Minoan civilisation here) sounds very much like ancient Sparta in its treatment of its youth: 'from boyhood they should grow up accustomed to arms and toils, so as to scorn heat, cold, marches over rugged and steep roads, and blows received in gymnasiums or regular battles.'[13] However, Greek geographer Strabo, writing in the first century BCE, maintains that the Cretans were the first to institute widespread child cruelty which was 'only perfected by the Spartans'.[14] Which is one in the eye to Lycurgus as the solo innovator of Spartan society.

'They have a peculiar custom in regard to love affairs,'[15] begins Strabo. Strabo, it should be noted, is writing about a Crete that existed many centuries before him; however, he is using as his source a Greek historian, Ephorus, who lived in the fourth century BCE and who he quotes directly. That Strabo has access to the writings of a contemporary to the Cretan customs gives his account more weight than many we have looked at. Although we shouldn't forget that Strabo is interpreting Ephorus' words through the eyes of a man living 500 years later, the equivalent of your twenty-first-century secondary school pupil reading Shakespeare's plays. The jokes in a Shakespeare comedy are lost on a modern audience because their context is lost, necessitating an enormous number of footnotes explaining why a particular line would have been funny half a millennia ago. Although even that is an assumption by the footnote writer that the audience who heard it in the context of the time didn't all groan or throw turnips at the actors responsible for such a horrendously unfunny gag. Strabo is interpreting and translating unfamiliar customs to his modern audience, something to bear in mind.

The peculiar custom Strabo goes on to describe is about as far removed as you can get from the mannered and carefully choreographed ritualised courtship we saw in Athens between *erastes* and *eromenos*. 'They win the objects of their love, not by persuasion, but by abduction.'[16] In Crete, the equivalent of the Athenian *erastes* tells the friends of his chosen boy that he plans to abduct him in three or four days' time, he even tells them where and then threatens them not to 'conceal the boy, or not to let him go forth by the appointed road'.[16] The friends are then made accomplices to this abduction: 'the friends pursue him and lay hold of him, though only in a very gentle way, thus satisfying the custom; and after that they cheerfully turn the boy over to him to lead away.'[17] It's worth stressing here that the boy at the centre of this 'mock' abduction has no idea it's going to happen, his consent has not been sought, and this is before we get to scenario B.

Scenario A, as described above, where the boys' friends cheerfully hand him over to an adult man who has taken a fancy to him, is all based on said adult male being worthy of the boy. To be worthy of the boy is quantified as being 'the boy's equal or superior in rank or other respects'.[18] Speculate away as to what those 'other respects' might be. In scenario B, where the adult male is considered not worthy, the friends do not 'cheerfully' hand over their friend to this strange man, they fight him off.

After a successful abduction, our scenario A, the boy is given gifts and then

> the abductor takes him away to any place in the country he wishes; and those who were present at the abduction follow after them, and after feasting and hunting with them for two months (for it is not permitted to detain the boy for a longer time), they return to the city. The boy is released after receiving as presents a military habit, an ox, and a drinkingcup.[19]

The heavily ritualised nature of this Cretan tradition, e.g. the gifts given, obscure that a boy has been taken away from his family home and forced to live with a strange man for two whole months.

Strabo makes it sound almost jolly, what with the hunting and feasting and the boy having his best pals with him the whole two months, but then we get this passage:

> Now the boy sacrifices the ox to Zeus and feasts those who returned with him; and then he makes known the facts about his intimacy with his lover, whether, perchance, it has pleased him or not, the law allowing him this privilege in order that, if any force was applied to him at the time of the abduction, he might be able at this feast to avenge himself and be rid of the lover.[20]

That there is a law in place for the abducted to gain recompense shows up that this wasn't all some cute old custom with play acting, boys were raped, and everyone was aware of that fact.

That a mock abduction had the potential to stray into nasty territory was likely due to the pressure placed on the adult male. 'It is disgraceful for those who are handsome in appearance or descendants of illustrious ancestors to fail to obtain lovers, the presumption being that their character is responsible for such a fate.'[21] Under such social pressure you can see how it could all go wrong and also accounts for the great honours the boy receives later, for as well as all the gifts his abductor has already showered upon him, he received 'honours; for in both the dances and the races they have the positions of highest honour, and are allowed to dress in better clothes than the rest, that is, in the habit given them by their lovers; and not then only, but even after they have grown to manhood, they wear a distinctive dress.'[22]

We could write this off as something we, thousands of years later, without being privy to the viewpoints of either abductor or abductee, cannot possibly understand. That we are not in a position to judge the norms of a society so far removed from our own. That perhaps it was all ritualistic and we are reading too much into it. But then we have these words of the contemporary Plato. 'The Cretans are said to have invented the tale of Zeus and Ganymede in order to justify their evil practices by the example of the Gods.'[23] Ganymede being a young boy that the king of the gods, Zeus, abducted in the guise of an eagle and forced the boy to be his cupbearer for ever more. Plato's words make it clear that other Greeks did not view the Cretans' practices as a harmless ritual, they recognised a darkness hiding underneath just as we do.

Elis

We know very little about Greek love and homosexuality in ancient Elis aside from it earned the tutting disapproval of both Plato and Cicero, which alone makes it worth taking a brief paragraph or two of examination.

In Plato's *Symposium*, one of the guests explains that in 'in Elis and Boeotia, and wherever people are not clever speakers, it has been simply decreed that the gratification of lovers is good, and no one, old or young, would suggest that it is a disgrace. This, I presume, is to save them the trouble of trying to persuade the young people, when they are such inadequate speakers.'[24] This is a burn of epic proportions on the Eleans and Boetians, clever speaking was what ancient Athens was all about, it's what Plato's *Symposium* was all about.

The likes of the Eleans weren't clever enough for Greek love Athenian style, where an *eromenos* was a prize to be won with gifts and seducing words and gave in to the *erastes*' sexual desires if he believed he had been given sufficient moral and intellectual improvement. The Eleans viewed sex as a positive and physically pleasurable activity that did not require the moral or intellectual improvement of either party. The barbarians!

Cicero's tutting disapproval is in the same vein as Plato's. 'To say nothing of the Eleans and Thebans, among whom lust is actually given free rein in the relations of free men.'[25] Although there is an important distinction here, Plato was an Athenian living in the fifth century BCE, Cicero is a Roman in the first century BCE – these are two very different cultures when it comes to attitudes to homosexuality. In Athens in the fifth century BCE, the *erastes* and the *eromenos* are both of the elite class, with the younger man required to be the passive partner in the relationship. Ancient Rome also considered age difference an important factor in same-sex relations, the younger partner again had to be the passive one. However, in Rome class played a larger role, it was socially unacceptable for an elite Roman man or boy to be the passive partner of another Roman male, it rendered him effeminate, unmanly and un-Roman: Romans were doers, they were the active, the penetrators, the rampaging across continent conquerors. Romans were dominant, never passive.

The only acceptable same-sex partner for an elite Roman male was someone lower in class, most likely a slave boy, because there were laws protecting freeborn boys. Greek love in any form, be it the elaborate mentorship of Athens or the simple acceptance of homosexuality in Elis, was an abomination to the Romans. You can tell how much they disapproved of it by the number of politicians and emperors who are slandered as having given in to an older man whilst in their youth. For example, Julius Caesar was said to have given in sexually to the King of Bithynia, later changing roles and supposedly buggering his great-nephew, Octavian. In ancient Greece, this tale could be spun as the greatest ever double act of *erastes* and *eromenos*, given that Octavian later morphs into Rome's first emperor Augustus; Caesar must have mentored him hard and well for him to achieve so much. In Rome both stories are slurs to be hurled for political capital. Cicero's disapproval is very much stressed on the 'free men' aspect of the Elean culture.

Lovers in arms? – Thebes

The inhabitants of Boeotia are cast alongside the Eleans for dubious sexual practices, so let us take a look at them, how do they compare? The city of Thebes, situated in Boeotia, was one of the more prominent of the Greek city states with a distinguished past that stretched back to the golden age when the heroes roamed the land finding golden fleeces, surviving labyrinths and scalping snake-haired gorgons. Thebes counted Oedipus amongst its kings, successfully repelled an attack by the magnificent seven (seven champions chosen by the King of Argos to destroy Thebes) and counted Heracles amongst its defenders. Politically Thebes maintained a stance of being somewhat unpredictable and unreliable.

Although Thebes had sent its army as back-up to the doomed 300 Spartans at the Battle of Thermopylae holding back the Persian invasion of 480 BCE, by the summer of 479 BCE, rather than holding back the Persian masses from invading Greece, we find the Thebans fighting with the invaders against a Greek defence they'd been a part of only a few months earlier.

During the Peloponnesian War, they sided with the Spartans they had both fought with and against during the Persian war. In the wake of helping the Spartans to victory in the Peloponnesian War, we find the Thebans refusing to recognise the resulting Spartan hegemony, delighting themselves in winding up the now dominant power in Greece and their supposed ally. According to Xenophon, Thebes refused to join a Spartan-led assault on Piraeus and 'persuading the Corinthians likewise not to join that campaign'.[26] They'd also decided they weren't going to take part in the Spartan king Agesilaus' war in Asia, had stopped the king from making a sacrifice at Aulis, 'and had cast from the altar the victims already offered'.[27] For such behaviour, the Spartans thought the Thebans insolent and in need of a good kick up the bum to remind them just who was the big cheese in Greece now Athens had been defeated.

This is a good illustration of how impossible the Greeks were, they really could not work together beyond an immediate necessity. You would have thought that, given Sparta's fearsome reputation in battle, the Thebans might have laid off the kicking over of altars and committed themselves to aiding their ally in battle when told to. But the Spartans weren't nearly as competent in battle as they liked to pretend, something the Thebans had been steadily testing. 'The Thebans too by always engaging singly in Boeotia with the Lacedaemonians, and by fighting battles with them, which though not important in themselves nevertheless afforded them much practice and training.'[28] Thebes was about to step into the limelight. Sparta's (dubious) reputation as an unstoppable military force and the power in Greece came to an end at the hands of an invigorated Theban army at the Battle of Leuctra in 371 BCE.

It is a great footnote in history, the counterpoint of the tale of those 300 Spartans who fought what they knew was a losing battle because of the commonality they felt for their fellow Greeks and a strong, ethical, moral sense of duty that had been beaten into them from childhood. Thebes became the new power in Greece by being fundamentally untrustworthy, they were not going to die defending anyone's hill, not even their own, if offered enough incentives by the other side. They were perversely both allied to Sparta and Athens at different points during the Peloponnesian War.

I am perhaps being unkind to the Thebans, Plutarch is much nicer about their national character in his biography of Pelopidas, the general who bested the Spartans and others in the fourth century BCE. 'The true reason for the superiority of the Thebans was their virtue, which led them not to aim their actions at glory or wealth, which are naturally attended by bitter envying and strife; on the contrary they were both filled from the beginning with a divine desire to see their country become most powerful and glorious.'[29] Plutarch, it's worth noting, was a native of Boeotia, which doesn't necessarily make him biased but does lend him to seeing Theban actions in a distinctly glowing light.

If you're wondering what this potted history of Thebes has to do with Greek love, the answer is everything because this invigorated Theban army had at its core what was called the Sacred Band; an elite fighting force made up of pairs of male lovers. Which takes us back once again to Plato's *Symposium*, at some point I will stop referencing this work but not yet... You'll recall Phaedrus' speech in which he talked about one of the benefits of Greek love being how it made you braver lest you be diminished in your lover's eyes. 'If there were only some way of contriving that a state or an army should be made up of lovers and their loves, they would be the very best governors of their own city, abstaining from all dishonour, and emulating one another in honour; and when fighting at each other's side, although a mere handful, they would overcome the world.'[30] This is pretty much exactly what Thebes had done, which eventually (although briefly) gave them hegemony over the other city states.

Plutarch has a naturally glowing example of what Phaedrus talks about. 'Pelopidas after receiving seven wounds in front, sank down upon a great heap of friends and enemies who lay dead together, but Epaminodas, although he thought him lifeless stood forth to defend his body and arms and fought desperately, single handed against many determined to die rather than leave Pelopidas lying there.'[31] Which is all very stirring and cinematic and what was at the heart of the Sacred Band. For as Plutarch says, 'tribesmen and clansmen make little account of tribesmen and clansmen in times of danger, whereas a band that is held together by the friendship of lovers is indissoluble.'[32]

Plutarch doesn't half dredge up stirring scenes from the history of the Sacred Band, such as when the band are slaughtered by the Macedonians and the victorious Philip is taken to see his dead enemies. 'Philip was surveying the dead, and stopped at the place where the three hundred were all lying … with their armour and mingled with one another he was amazed on learning that this was the band of lovers and beloved, burst into tears.'[33] There is something here in the Greek national character that prizes love above everything else, so much so that it moves the hardened one-eyed general Philip of Macedon to tears.

I get it, the horror of being in battle with your other half, the terror of something happening to them constantly on your mind and then the something terrible does happen and you witness it first-hand. That desperate pain as you see your lover fall and then the sheer fury that courses through your veins at those responsible. Yes, I can see how that could create an elite fighting force, although for us to believe that both you and I have to put aside everything we have learnt in our collective lives about relationships.

The ancient Greeks may have lionised both beauty and love as transcendent, nay divine qualities to be admired and worshipped, but we all know that somebody has to put the bins out, remember to buy a pint of milk on their way home from work and desist from doing that super irritating thing with their nostrils. I find it very hard to believe, actually impossible to believe that some of that everyday mundane stuff of life did not find its way into the ranks. Some of the sacred Theban Band had to be standing, shields raised, watching the enemy advance, hearts pounding in their chests, gearing up for the brutal battle to come when they happened to glance upon the man standing next to them, their partner/lover and thought, 'God, I hope you die.'

For all we know, those dead Thebans discovered by Philip of Macedon, their limbs and armour intermingling, were not the victims of the Macedonian onslaught into Greece but rather a bloody release of tension after weeks spent sharing a tent with a man who eats with his mouth open and whose toes are way too hairy.

The paedophile poet of Sardis

The author of *Love, Sex and Marriage in Ancient Greece*, who we saw earlier defining Athenian-style Greek love as 'the spiritual affection and admiration for a boy'[34] whilst stating that we should not confuse this in any way with child abuse, defines what he refers to as 'pederasty' and which I've termed 'Greek love' as occurring in a particular time frame. 'Pederasty is a phenomenon that appeared approximately in the middle of the sixth century and flourished roughly until the end of the fourth century BCE.'[35] There is a reason I suspect the author chooses this cut-off point, because later sources, particularly poetry, comprehensively explode any notion that relations between adult men and youths were spiritually uplifting and mentoring.

Straton of Sardis was a Greek living under Roman rule in the second century CE and he was a strong adherent to the man/boy love ethos that NAMBLA are so expressive on. We know of Straton's predilections because he documented his boy-crazy life in many, many poems. 'I really like pale boys and I also love them honey coloured and golden too, although I am taken with ebony ones. Nor do I overlook hazel eyes. But I exceedingly love boys with lustrous dark eyes.'[36]

He admires 'the dusty grime of a gymnasium boy'[37] and he delights 'in the prime of a boy of twelve, but one of thirteen is much more desirable. He who is fourteen is a still sweeter flower of the Loves, and one who is just beginning his fifteenth year is yet more delightful. The sixteenth year is that of the gods, and as for the seventeenth it is not for me.'[38]

As you can tell, Straton spends a lot of time checking boys out, including 'my neighbour's quite tender young boy'.[39] If this sounds creepy, it decidedly is, as shown by the rest of this poem: '[He] provokes me not a little, and laughs in no novice manner to show me that he is willing. But he is not more than twelve years old. Now the unripe grapes are unguarded; when he ripens there will be watchmen and stakes.' Watchmen and stakes to keep the likes of Straton away.

Another poem of Straton's make this abuse all the clearer:

> Once a wrestling-master, taking advantage of the occasion, when he was giving a lesson to a smooth boy, forced him to kneel down, and set about working on his middle stroking the berries with one hand. But by chance the master of the house came, wanting the boy. The teacher threw him quickly on his back, getting astride of him and grasping him by the throat.[40]

In Sardis in the second century CE, Straton is not waxing lyrical on his favourite subject amongst his chums à la Plato's *Symposium*, he's being attacked by teachers and glared at with suspicion by parents. He's a predator, not a courting *erastes*. Boy, how things have changed.

A final note

This chapter and its predecessor have been heavy on same-sex relationships, but light on the word 'homosexual' or 'homosexuality', in fact those two words only appear nineteen times out of a possible 12,956 words. There is a reason for this. What we have looked at over the course of 12,000+ words is not homosexuality, at least not what we would call homosexuality today in the twenty-first century. To us to be homosexual is to be attracted exclusively to members of your own sex; this does not exist in ancient Greece as a concept. Every Athenian man who splashed love notes on a vase to his *eromenos* and stuck his erect penis between his thighs would later be married to a woman. The same is true of the other city states we have looked at like Sparta and Thebes, the Sacred Band was sacred only when it came to fighting; once the battling was over, Theban men were expected to marry Theban women and make little Thebans. The idea of a loving long-term relationship between people of the same sex does not exist in ancient Greece. You see this just as clearly in mythology, yes, Ganymede is Zeus' cup boy in the eternity of the heavens of Olympia, but Zeus is married to Hera who he is unthinkingly unfaithful to with many, many women.

This may surprise you because you might have heard Alexander the Great being touted as an early gay icon because of his longstanding relationship with his best friend, Hephaestion. However, you'll be hard pressed to find any actual mention of Alexander and Hephaestion being lovers in any ancient source, the closest you will find is lines such as Arrian's description of Hephaestion as being 'the man who was dearest to him in the whole world'.[41] Alexander's grief at the death of Hephaestion was seen to be excessive, which is the context for Arrian's line, it's a justification for that display of emotion from the military genius, but nowhere does it explicitly say they were lovers. It is our modern thinking dragging out a subtext that might not actually be there. Alternatively, it might, we have no way of knowing.

Even if Alexander and Hephaestion were long-term lovers, Alexander certainly wasn't what we would class as homosexual. When introduced to the Persian princess Roxana, later his wife, 'They also say that no sooner did Alexander see her than he fell in love with her.'[42] Bisexuality is the most we can claim for Alexander the Great, although nowhere is it attested that he claimed it for himself.

What we find in ancient Greece is something that is not homosexuality, nor is it straight-up paedophilia as we understand that, it is something entirely different that does not exist in our society and that we don't have an English word for. I've used the term 'Greek love', as stolen from Oscar Wilde, to describe it. Our society has laws against Greek love. The Sexual Offences Act 2003 has an entire section dedicated to abuses by people in positions of trust; it defines a position of trust as, 'a person looks after persons under 18 if he is regularly involved in caring for, training, supervising or being in sole charge of such persons'.[43] 'Caring, training and supervising' is exactly the duties of the Athenian *erastes*. The Sexual Offences Act of 2003 also includes the over-18s in its protection from those abuses of trust.

This, I think, is why we find it so hard to get our heads around Greek love, because it is stepping over the boundaries of what we see as a sacred relationship, so sacred we put it in our laws, that between teacher and pupil, mentor and mentee.

Chapter 7

Boys Will Be Boys: The Symposium

Symposium is another one of those Greek-invented words that pepper the English language. The *Cambridge Dictionary* defines a *symposium* as 'an occasion at which people who have a great knowledge of a particular subject meet in order to discuss a matter of interest'.[1] Which sounds deadly dull, and suggests to me a crowd of anoraked men, their cheeks flushing red with fury, as they loudly debate whether the fabric used on the London Underground's Victoria Line seats is superior upholstery to that used on the Central Line. Apologies to any London Underground enthusiasts who uniquely combine their love of railways and trains with a keen interest in ancient sexuality, we should definitely hold a *symposium* exploring that intersectionality.

Thankfully the ancient Greek *symposium* was quite unlike our modern usage of the word which places it in the realm of an academia understood by few.[2] The word *symposium* translates from the Greek as 'drinking together' and that's exactly what the Greeks did, they drank. Forget your clever people and their niche interests getting together to make their subject even more impenetrable to the layman, wipe clean from your mind all images of lecture theatres and PowerPoint presentations that seemingly last for hours, for they have nothing in common with an ancient Greek *symposium*. In ancient Greece, a *symposium* was a piss-up.

At its most basic level, the ancient Greek *symposium* involved a group of men gathering at one of their homes for an evening of conversation, a few nibbles, some form of entertainment and a steady supply of wine to keep the atmosphere light. If you're thinking that sounds all very civilised, think again. 'Very often, if not always, the symposium ended up in an orgy.'[3] This claim by Nikolaos A. Vrisimtzis, whose credentials include degrees from both the Sorbonne and the National University of Athens, is not lightly deployed.

The host of a *symposium* would direct his guests to an area of his house known as the *andron* or men's room which is fitting because only men could attend. Wives, daughters, granddaughters, favourite nieces and that weird but sexy female cousin of yours were not invited, even though they might only be a few hundred feet away in the same house. This already sets the scene for what a *symposium* was and very much wasn't, as does the one class of women who were permitted to attend a *symposium*, the *hetairai*. The *hetairai* were what was considered high-class prostitutes.

The *hetairai*, although not strictly guests, were allowed to add to the ongoing conversation, courted for a wit and charm that would enhance the atmosphere of the *symposium*. The only other women in attendance were also there purely for the men's enjoyment; flute girls, dancing girls and harp playing girls were all forms of entertainment offered at a *symposium*. They are also all graphically depicted on Greek pottery, having lain down their instrument, at least temporarily, to provide a very different form of entertainment for the guests; one that required a different kind of plucking and fewer clothes.

The *hetairai* might find themselves on the guest list for their conversational skills, but they too were expected to entertain the men sexually; if we are to believe the depictions reproduced on pottery this could involve multitudes of men simultaneously. The images that have survived of *symposia* are some of the most extreme to be found on ancient Greek pottery, they involve chains of men and women engaging in oral, vaginal and anal sex, often all at the same time. Which is as far removed as you can get from the image we have of bushy bearded Greek men gently moulding and cradling Western civilisation in their hands, ready to hand it over to us. Those geniuses that so inspired Byron and Shelley were the same geniuses who held sex parties within the hearing of their wives and daughters and then celebrated it on crockery.

We have literary evidence too for Greek *symposia* being all-out sex parties. A certain Phrynion took his personal hetairai 'everywhere with him to dinners where there was drinking and making her a partner in his revels; and he had intercourse with her openly whenever and wherever he wished, making his privilege a display to the onlookers'.[4]

However, not every *symposium* was necessarily an all-out orgy of the worst of male drunken behaviour inflicted upon women who had no choice but to partake. Although it is staggering to think that such events did occur in a house where but a few hundred feet away were the host's female relations. There is something deeply disturbing and revealing about how ancient Greek men thought and treated both the women they supposedly most cared for and 'other' women. This is something we shall be picking apart in more detail in later chapters.

The two fullest accounts we have of a *symposium* come from Plato and Xenophon, neither of which is a drunken orgy. Although in the case of Plato's *symposium* this appears to be because most of the guests attended another *symposium* the previous night that quite possibly could have been heavy on the orgytastic and they all got absolutely hammered. With thundering hangovers they forgo the fun elements of a standard *symposium*, booze and birds, and instead launch into what you would think was less than kind to their pounding heads and dry tongues, an extended philosophical discussion on the nature of love. This goes on for many, many lines as the guests who include a comic playwright, a physician, a poet, a legal expert and the philosopher Socrates make a series of speeches about love that'll keep academics happily pulling them apart for millennia and inspire Oscar Wilde into some really quite dreadful behaviour.

These deep philosophical musings are interrupted by Athenian bad boy Alcibiades, who turns up roaring drunk to this sober talkfest and immediately livens it up by 'appearing at the door crowned with a massive garland of ivy and violets, his head flowing with ribands'. He too gives a speech on the nature of love despite being at a great disadvantage to his fellow speakers by way of being completely off his face.

Socrates is also a guest of the *symposium* that Xenophon describes and it's a better read and clearly a much better party than Plato's. At Xenophon's do we get some proper entertainment rather than a series of long speeches; there's a flute girl, a dancing girl with additional acrobatic talents and who can juggle whilst being rotated on a pottery wheel and a handsome boy dancer who always played the cither. A cither, if anyone is wondering, resembles a tiny, more practically portable harp.

One of the guests, Philip, suffers from the delusion that he is an amusing man and attempts to inject what he believes are witticisms: 'finding he did not excite any laughter he showed himself for some time considerably vexed.'[5]

Awkward. But not so awkward as to completely crush Philip's spirit, which is a shame because his next attempt at comedy falls even flatter. We've all been that person at the party/work conference/down the pub desperately wanting to be part of a fun conversation and in our eagerness have dropped in a line that inadvertently kills that fun conversation dead. In that moment, with all eyes upon you, your only and sincerely felt wish is that one of those sinkhole things you saw on the internet the other week would open up beneath your feet and swallow you whole. Philip has a similar reaction at Xenophon's *symposium*. 'He stopped while the dinner was in full swing, covered his cloak with his head and lay down his head on his couch.'[6] Talk about drama queens! Philip is clearly a man who needs the centre of attention to be on him, for good or ill.

There are no long speeches in Xenophon's *symposium* but rather a more quick-witted exchange of ideas and philosophy on what each of the guests take pride in, where men harbour their righteousness, the nature of beauty and love and various other bits and bobs of chit chat.

Although both Xenophon and Plato's parties lack the degeneracy of some accounts of *symposia*, their evenings follow the exact same structure: firstly, the guests arrive and there is chit chat over nibbles and wine, next hymns are sung to the gods and a libation poured in their honour, then comes the entertainment, accompanied by more drinking and more chit chat. Within this structure, Xenophon and Plato present evenings that are extremely different in tone, despite Socrates being a guest at both events, and the mutual aim of inventing these *symposia* to push Socrates' flavour of philosophy, of which both Plato and Xenophon were fanboys.

The reason these two *symposia* are so different and indeed why any other two *symposia* differed from each other is down to the *Symposiarch*, the host of the *symposium*. It is the *Symposiarch* who sets the tone of the evening and he does so by every choice he makes about his event: the guest list, the entertainments on offer and the wine that will be served.

Archaeological evidence suggests that a *symposium* room contained a maximum of nine couches. With two people to each couch, this made a guest list of fewer than twenty, which makes for a select and selected list, cruelly exposing exactly where you stand with your fellow citizens – outside on the street listening to the jollity occurring beyond a door that's not opening for you.

Another important component of a *symposium* was wine. Lots of wine. It wouldn't have been much of a drinking party without wine. One important difference from the drinking of wine in our time is that the Greeks adulterated their wine with water: ordinarily three or four parts water to one part wine, which was mixed in a large vessel known as a krater. Although it should be noted that this watered-down wine in no way lessened the level of inebriation of the invited guests. One of the key decisions that the host of any *symposium* had to decide was how many kraters of wine he would be mixing for the evening and the proportions of that mixture. This single act very much signposted what sort of an evening was planned; convivial discussion or a falling down drunk, throwing up kind of night.

So we have wine, we have women in the shape of the *hetairai*, what else did well-planned *symposia* require? Entertainment, that's what! This could be the sexual talents of the *hetairai* or else musicians and dancers, such as Xenophon notes. Aside from these provided distractions, the other entertainment provided was so very ancient Greek, conversation – a *symposium* was a place for men to talk. Big subjects were covered, deep philosophical conversations on the nature of love and mankind and the markers of a civilisation. And then everyone had sex with the attending prostitutes or with the serving wine boys or with each other. There is no similarity between a *symposium* and the modern dinner party, unless I'm being invited to all the wrong parties.

As noted earlier, there is special homeware associated with a *symposium*, wine coolers, kraters for mixing in the water, cups to drink from. This is crockery chosen especially for hosting *symposia* and not crockery that was used elsewhere in the house for domestic meals. Of course, we can never truly know if this was indeed the case, but I think it's a fair deduction that Mrs Greek Wife wasn't serving up the kiddies' bedtime milk in cups depicting prostitutes being penetrated by multiple men in multiple orifices or naked satyrs balancing wine kraters on their erect penises. The illustrations on *symposia* crockery are both wild and anatomically impossible in several cases.

Many of the filthiest illustrations are to be found at the bottom of a cup as a pleasant surprise for those that drained their wine. We also find drinking vessels that you can only drink from by placing your mouth around the penis-shaped spout. Who knew that pottery could be so rich and filthy a topic? But like the strength of the wine, the inclusion of the *hetairai* and the other entertainments on offer, the rude cups set the tone for the evening.

Even though Xenophon's account of a *symposium* is a literary vehicle for him to deliver the thoughts of his hero, Socrates, it nonetheless gives us an insight into the nature of the event, it's no casual dinner party, that's for sure. In Xenophon's account, Callias is hosting a *symposium* to honour the victory of a certain Autolycus in the *pankration*. On spotting Socrates and his chums, Callias immediately offers them up an invitation, persuading them with the line, 'If you favour me with your company I will prove to you that I am a person of some consequence.'[7]

This really sums up what is at the heart of a *symposium*, it's about showing yourself to be 'of some consequence' or a good citizen in other words. Think about the layout of the *symposium* room, the couches all face inwards so that everyone is on display to everyone else, including in Xenophon's *symposium*, star guest Autolycus, whose display nobody can stop looking at. 'The beauty of Autolycus compelled everyone to look at him. And again, there was not one of the onlookers who did not feel his soul strangely stirred by the boy, some of them grew quieter than before, others even assumed some kind of a pose.'[8] You do have to wonder how Autolycus has maintained his good looks given his recent *pankration* victory, what no black eye, broken fingers and throttle marks round his throat?

When the uninvited Philip turns up, the host Callias 'cast a glance at Autolycus, obviously trying to make out what he had thought'.[9] It is so very important to Callias how he is seen by his fellow citizens, to prove that he is worthy of their company and his own position in society. Throw a good *symposium* and you'll be the talk of the agora the next day, badly mismatch your guests with the entertainments, or provide too little in the way of refreshments, then you'll still be the talk of the agora the next day but in a hushed whisper, eyes averted way. You'll likely find your next *symposium* invites turned down by some of the great and the good and the influential. If Callias duffs up his evening, no gorgeous *pankration* winner is going to cross his threshold ever again.

We've talked about the sort of crockery that was especially chosen to match the tone of the *symposium* but there is one vessel I have not mentioned yet, and for a change it has nothing to do with what is depicted on the outside of it (hardcore pornographic or otherwise), but rather it's shape. It's called a kylix, and it is the equivalent of our wine glass. See Image 32 for an example of a kylix.

It doesn't look much like a drinking vessel; it looks more like a dessert dish, being narrow in depth with wide handles either side. If you have ever tried to drink from a cereal bowl, and which of us hasn't at some point in our life during a petty house dispute on who's turn it is to do the washing up, you'll know that this inevitably results in a spillage of some sort. It certainly isn't graceful, and I wouldn't recommend you attempt it in front of an audience, particularly one you want to think well of you. Which begs the question why on earth is the kylix the drinking vessel of choice at a *symposium*? It's not as if the Greeks didn't know how to make cups, we have thousands of examples that they did, so why? It is another test, another way of proving you are a proper citizen for only the most refined, skilled and worthy of men can drink from the kylix without it pouring down the side of their faces whilst lying reclined.

Showing off, whether it be your finely gym-toned body or the very attractive *eromenos* you've won over or your ability to make an impromptu philosophical argument on the subject of love and even drinking from a cup that clearly is not built for that function is a very ancient Greek trait.

Chapter 8
Penises

I debated for some time on what to call this chapter. One contender for the title was: 'Ithyphallic Imagery in Ancient Greek Culture', which follows the well-trodden academic path of hiding in plain sight fascinating information using obscure words that only other academics understand, it's the opposite of clickbait: it's a scroll past. This chapter is about penises; it is about statues of gods with rigid erect penises, vase paintings of freaky birds with penises for heads, depictions of satyrs surprised by their penises and penises themselves, depicted with wings, feet and, yes, penises of their own. There is no escaping those one-eyed snakes in this chapter, consider the title a disclaimer for any readers who suffer from phallophobia, that is a fear of penises.

Before we embark on our penile tour, we need to first talk terminology. Hopefully we all know what a penis is, if not go find a biology book, have a flick through the diagrams and then rejoin us enlightened. Alongside penis, which has already been used ten times in our first two paragraphs, the other word you will find liberally scattered throughout this chapter like contraceptives in a brothel (or so I imagine, do find me on social media and correct me if I'm wrong) is phallus. Phallus can be used as an alternative to the word penis, along with many other words, some of which are probably now popping into your head uninvited. If you have a spare ten minutes I'd recommend heading for the website of the prestigious American Stanford University which hosts what presumably is a research paper by one of its students; a three-page dossier of slang words for penis.[1] It must be a very American-centric list or perhaps it's because I'm a woman, but most of these words I've never heard in general usage, which I'm thankful for. The man who describes his appendage as the ground squirrel, the sticky grenade or the Lincoln Memorial is the man whose number I am going to block on my phone.

Phallus in ancient Greece refers specifically to an erect penis, which you will see as readily depicted in images from the time as its flaccid counterpart and in contexts we, as twenty-first-century humans, boggle at. Notably the phallus has strong connections to religion and is a religious symbol. Another word we may stumble across in this chapter is ithyphallic, which is a way of referring collectively to objects and images that possess phallic qualities.

Ancient Greece is an ithyphallic society: big time. Forget the nudie statues and our naked gymnasium bunnies of earlier chapters, the penis is a far bigger topic because the phallus/penis was to be found everywhere in ancient Greece. There's no pretending it wasn't, not when a key Greek festival involved not only the waving around of models of erect penises by participants but also the baking of special penis-shaped cakes. At the other end of the penis scale, the island of Delos hosts the remains of a temple dedicated to Dionysius, the entrance to which is flanked by two phalluses. Sadly, only the testicles and bottom of the shaft of these two mighty penises survive but the size of the surviving fragments lead us to conclude that these were big knobs, very big knobs indeed (see Image 34). If any chapter will convince you how different ancient Greeks and ancient Greek society were to us and our society, this is that chapter.

The divine penis

Here in the twenty-first century, we think of ourselves as liberated, confident and open when talking about sex compared to previous generations, and this is generally thought of as a good thing. Generally, but not completely, because there are many who believe these more sexually liberated times are not a good thing at all but instead damaging to society. There are strong arguments on both sides of this debate and it's one that has been raging since the 1960s upended the rigid social order and morals that preceded it.

Heading into the world of social media, reasoned debates are much harder to come by, outrage and offence not so much. There are very few people on social media who are not upset about something and determined to recruit others to their side. One event recently that seemed to upset a great many keyboard complainers was the opening ceremony of the 2024 Olympics in Paris. One irate viewer, on social media platform X, described the opening ceremony as being a vile celebration of fetishised male cross-dressing, freakishness, brutal violence and satanic themes. This criticism makes the Paris opening ceremony sound way more interesting than it was.

Compared to the opening ceremony of the annual Athenian festival, the Great Dionysia, the Paris Olympics with its hint of a threesome and fashion-parading drag queens appears subtle and tame. At no point during those rain-soaked hours in France was there 'a phallus procession; a penis parade of drunk men carrying large cocks and shouting obscenities as they cavorted through town'.[2] More's the pity, it would have made it far more entertaining viewing.

This penis parade was part of the procession that followed a wagon transporting a statue of the god Dionysius through the streets of Athens to the theatre that bore the god's name. Dionysius was the god of wine and merriment, but also on his CV of divine responsibilities were ecstasy, insanity, dance, fertility, orchards, fruit and theatre. It's a mixed bag of attributes for sure, juicy apples on the one hand, losing your mind on the other.

The Bacchae by Euripides depicts the darker side of Dionysius, it is a play you walk away from having read or seen performed with glazed eyes and a troubled soul. The plot of *The Bacchae* is set in Thebes, a city Dionysius and his entourage of high-spirited followers have decided to visit. This does not please a certain Pentheus who, hearing rumours about Dionysius' jolly antics, decides that he does not like the sound of them one bit. 'It so happens I've been away from Thebes, but I hear about disgusting things going on, here in the city – women leaving home to go to silly Bacchic rituals, cavorting there in mountain shadows, with dances honouring some upstart god, this Dionysus, whoever he may be.'[3]

Pentheus gives out orders to capture the 'effeminate' stranger and 'tie him up and bring him here for judgment, a death by stoning. That way he'll see his rites in Thebes come to a bitter end.'[4] Greek myths are awash with people who bitterly regret an off-the-cuff remark that could possibly be seen as disrespectful to a god; Pentheus is openly denying that Dionysius is a god and treating him as a mortal man. This is a heinous crime, one worthy of a heinous punishment.

Dionysius' vengeance is dark indeed, he sends the women of Thebes into a frenzy of insanity. No longer in possession of their minds, the Theban women form a murderous mob who turn on Pentheus. Surrounded by the crazed women, Pentheus is literally pulled to pieces. 'Literally' is a word frequently misused, it is not here. The hapless and indeed helpless Pentheus' limbs are torn off by the women. Included in this killer crowd is Pentheus' own mother, Agave, on whom her son's pleading has no effect. Her sanity taken by Dionysius, she

> grabbed her son's arm, stepped on his shoulder blade and ripped his arm clean off his body ... Bits of his flesh were strewn about everywhere. Some up against the rough rocks others so deep in the shrubs of the forest that it was impossible to find them all. And his poor head! His mother happened to take a hold of it. She stuck it at the end of her thyrsus and now carries it around the mountain's paths.[5]

Dionysius was not a god to mess with and I can quite understand why Athens should feel the need each year to honour him, if only to make him feel loved enough not to inflict such brutal madness upon their womenfolk and create one hell of a bloody mess to mop up in the agora. Although the origin story of how the Great Dionysia festival came to be held in Athens has nothing to do with crazy women ripping off people's arms, thankfully.

The crime that preceded Pentheus' decapitated head being stuck on the end of a pole had been refusing to recognise the divinity of Dionysius. Athens' crime against Dionysius falls on the milder side, the people of Athens had not shown enough reverence to a statue of Dionysius that had been brought into the city. Not that Dionysius wasn't annoyed by this, he was, but not so annoyed he created a murderous mob of women to rip the statue-disrespecting citizens to pieces. Instead, he inflicted quite a different punishment on the men of Athens who he singled out by infecting them en masse with an itchy, red, sore and thoroughly unpleasant disease of the penis.

It's no rampaging mob of mad women intent on reducing them into chunks of bloody flesh, true, but it still wasn't very nice for the men. It wasn't very nice for their wives either, because who wants their husband under their feet all day, scratching at his groin and complaining? Clearly something had to be done to placate Dionysius and heal the collective penises of Athens. Pisistratus, who was the ruler of a pre-democratic Athens at this time,[6] knew just what was needed to make the god happy again, a jolly festival!

And so, from itchy penises was born the Great Dionysia festival. Although the main focus of the festival was a literary competition, the origins of this celebration were not forgotten and were reflected in the opening ceremony with the great statue of Dionysius pulled through the streets, followed on its route through the city by a parade of phallus bearers.

There is quite a lot to unpick here. Although the itchy penises are mentioned with frequency as the origin of the Great Dionysia, you will be hard pressed to find the original source of the story. This lack of an original source makes me highly suspicious that this is a tale invented in hindsight to explain why the Athenians have an annual parade where the citizens hold aloft penises of various sizes. On the other hand, it's bizarre enough a tale to be fully believable set against the sheer bonkersness of Greek mythology which includes, as one small example, a woman having sex with a swan. That this swan is Zeus in animal disguise does not in any way lessen that the woman, Leda, has sex with a bird, an image which inspired many works of art across the ages, and understandable questions about how anatomically possible such a union would be. So let us go along with the itchy penis disease story, whilst secretly wondering whether it's a clever defence for that time everyone got the clap off that one prostitute and had to explain it to their wives. Onwards with the penis parade!

At the front of the parade, behind the wagon carrying Dionysius, were the elite of Athenian society. One of their members was given the honour of holding a golden basket of fruit, the less honoured of the elite followed him carrying wine skins or loaves of bread, the staples of a feast. Following the foremost citizens of the *polis* were the people known as *metics*, these were residents of the city who were not citizens and who therefore could not play any part in the public life of the *polis*, such as voting in the assembly or holding any public position. The world's first democracy was distinctly undemocratic in our understanding of the word, it was an exclusive and excluding club. *Metics* were important to Athens, however, because somebody had to be involved in trade and building up the material wealth of the city whilst the citizens worked on building up the intellectual wealth that would make them the envy of the world.

In this opening procession of the Dionysia, the *metics* carried basins filled with honeycomb and cakes, their womenfolk accompanying them carrying water jugs. After the *metics* came the *ephebes*, those young men in military training, escorting the bull that would be sacrificed in honour of the god. Following the *ephebes* and their bull it was time to bring on the penises!

We have an account of this part of the parade from a play by Aristophanes called *The Acharnians*, in which the head of the household, Dicaeopolis, instructs, 'Xanthias, walk behind the basket-bearer and hold the phallus well erect; I will follow, singing the Phallic hymn; thou, wife, look on from the top of the terrace.'[7] Dicaeopolis' wife must watch from the terrace because married elite women were not allowed to partake in the phallus parade.

Dicaeopolis would have joined the groups of men walking along carrying aloft phalluses, singing hymns and shouting obscenities. Or, as the footnote to the translation of *The Acharnians* I am using describes the parade, 'the phallophori crowned with violets and ivy and their faces shaded with green foliage, sang improvised airs, called "Phallics," full of obscenity and suggestive "double entendres."'[8] Like I said, the Paris Olympic Opening Ceremony was tame in comparison, and dare I say it, boring.

The procession, phalluses and all, would culminate at the theatre of Dionysius where the god would gratefully receive his sacrificial bull and pile of penises. Opening ceremony completed, the main focus of the Great Dionysia could commence, the literary competition.

There were three categories of play that could be entered into the Dionysia festival: comedy, tragedy and satyr plays. The competition was fierce and produced works that astonishingly are still performed 2,500 years after they were written, plays by the likes of Sophocles, Aeschylus and Euripides. We know these three best for their tragedies; Sophocles was the author of *Oedipus Rex*, *Antigone*, *Ajax* and *Electra* amongst many others. Aeschylus gave the world *Prometheus Unbound* and *The Persians*, whilst Euripides produced *The Trojan Women* and *The Bacchae*. These three titans of Greek literature who bequeathed to us plays of such power and depth also authored numerous satyr plays, satyrs you'll remember are those chubby little fellows with furry legs, a tail and a permanent stiffy.

It doesn't quite fit, does it? That the writer of *Oedipus Rex*, a towering tale of hubris and of destiny preordained, whose finale has the heroine hanging herself and the hero gouging out his own eyes, also penned plays about horny satyrs. But he did, we know he did because the rules of the Great Dionysia competition stated that each playwright had to enter into the competition three tragic plays and one satyr play.

Of the plays entered into the Great Dionysia, we have been left with but a small selection of the total output. Sophocles, for example, is said to have written a whopping 120 plays, of which only seven survive in completion. It is perhaps not entirely surprising that of all the satyr plays that were ever written we have only one full play. I mean it's slightly odd, some might say suspicious that we have seven full Sophocles tragedies, seven surviving Aeschylus tragedies, three full surviving Euripides tragedies, eleven surviving Aristophanes comedies but only one full satyr play. It raises a lot of questions about how we come to have the literature we have, why some works have survived to the modern day and others did not, and why did they not?

These are important questions; however, we are going to daintily skip past all of them, because it's too big a subject for my meagre word count. Let us just blame some monk in a gloomy, sinister-looking monastery in fourteenth-century Germany for tossing scrolls of satyr plays into the fire because he didn't find them funny and move on. The sole fully intact survivor of its genre, the satyr play, *The Cyclops*, was a play written by the same guy who wrote the extremely bloody *The Bacchae*, Euripides.

The theatrical phallus

Euripides was the author of such weighty, and still frequently performed, plays as *Medea*: woman murders her own children to spite their unfaithful father, *Hecuba*: woman seeks revenge for the death of her son by blinding his murderer and killing all his sons, and the aforementioned *The Bacchae*: woman driven mad by a god rips her own son to pieces with her bare hands. I'm no Sigmund Freud but I'm strongly getting the impression that Euripides was a tiny bit frightened by women. It may be connected, it may very well not be connected, but as an aside Euripides was married twice and neither marriage went terribly well, with both of his wives taking lovers. I'm not saying his unhappy marriages influenced his plays, their plots are taken from Greek mythology and were already well-established stories, but I can see that writing certain scenes could have a cathartic effect on the inwardly enraged. There's also this tart exchange in an Aristophanes' play that features Euripides as a character.

> EURIPIDES: That is precisely what makes me tremble; the women have plotted my ruin, and to-day they are to gather in the Temple of Demeter to execute their decision.
>
> MNESILOCHUS: What have they against you?
>
> EURIPIDES: Because I mishandle them in my tragedies.
>
> MNESILOCHUS: By Poseidon, you would seem to have thoroughly deserved your fate.[9]

Euripides' satyr play *The Cyclops* does not continue any cathartic mass murdering, it contains such lines as '*Indicates his phallus*. Hahaha! One drink and a man can make this thing stand upright! Straight up! Upright and uptight! Hahahaha! One drink and a man can grab a woman's breast, enjoy a woman's shrub!'[10] And stage directions added in for clarity for future performers in the play, such as this one: 'more screams for a few seconds, then a short pause before Cyclops is heard belching, laughing heartily ... and farting.'[11] It's really not the sort of play that you could see Fiona Shaw and Simon Russell Beale scooping up Olivier awards from for their collection.

Ancient Greek comedies were populist entertainment that held a mirror up to Athenian society, lampooning the great and the good who had to suck it up like a Hollywood roast. Politicians Pericles and Cleon, playwrights Euripides and Aeschylus, and philosopher Socrates were all the targets of comedic plays. It was likely needed, a collective stepping back from the seriousness of the times and the seriousness of the men of the times and having a good laugh at their pomposity and actions.

There are several important differences in how ancient Greeks staged their plays compared to how we stage them today. Firstly, the actors would all have been male, even for female roles, and secondly all the actors would be wearing masks. This fundamentally changes the nature of acting in the ancient world as opposed to the modern; without being able to use your face to convey emotion, be it despair or laughter, and performing in outdoor theatres to a back row many metres away without any modern sound equipment, ancient acting had to be much more physical, more pronounced, more exaggerated, bigger.

That went for the costumes too. With male actors playing female characters, the audience had to clear which gender was which whether they had front-row seats or were sitting in the crappier seats right at the top rung of the theatre. Comedy was where this distinction was made the most obvious, for reasons that will become apparent. We know what type of masks and costumes comedy actors wore from depictions on vases. Here we see actors wearing grotesquely ugly-faced masks with noticeable pointed beards. Bodies were padded to look bigger (yes, the fat guy being the butt of lazy humour does instead stretch back that far) with particular emphasis on the stomach and buttocks, because again, well, comedy. The padding was held in place by the leotard-style garment that the actors wore and attached to this leotard was the leather phallus that was mentioned in Euripides' satyr play. Above this fake phallus was a tuft of fake pubic hair. This costume defines Greek comedy so that no one is going to accidentally think they're watching a tragedy. Although Sophocles' *Oedipus Rex* might have been given an extra layer of poignancy had the body part that had most caused Oedipus' plight been on full display to the audience the entire length of the play.

It's worth remembering the opening chapter of this book where we looked at the perfection of the male body personified by the statue of the Doryphoros. The costume of the comedy actor is the opposite of the perfect body of our Doryphoros statue, flabby, fleshy and with a penis that was not fashionably small and compact, signposting that these characters are there to be laughed at. See Images 37 and 38 for some examples of comic actors in costume.

A costume that consists of a flabby, floppy penis is a whole lake of inspiration for the comedy playwright to go fishing in. Greek comedy is not subtle, although there remains the possibility that it's packed full of subtle gags we can't recognise because we don't share the cultural baggage of the ancient Greeks. There are certainly satirical jabs at politicians and the world they have created, one in which the Peloponnesian War dragged ever onwards, but there is also an abundance of knob gags in Greek comedy. I mean you have it right there as a prop, why wouldn't you use it for cheap laughs?

We only have words on a page so we can never be sure what lines had the ancient Greeks crying with laughter and which fell flat as a toddler on an ice rink. We also don't have specific directions for the actors – translators and performers have taken their cues from the spoken lines of the characters, which helpfully lack subtlety. The sheer number of knob gags, both spoken and implied visually, and the various scenarios and plots they are squeezed into suggests they were a popular and expected part of any Greek comedy play.

Unfortunately, most of the winning comedic plays from the Great Dionysia have somehow got lost between then and now (damn that German monk!). Although there remains the possibility that some academic in a forgotten corridor of an esteemed university has stashed the lot in a safe, hidden behind a bust of Plato to preserve the reputation of the ancient Greeks as men of wisdom and gravitas. Unfortunately for that academic, but fortunately for us, we do have eleven full plays of Aristophanes, a quarter of his known output. We know that he was the victor of at least one of the Great Dionysia competitions and three times at the festival of Lenaia, another Athenian event dedicated to Dionysius which was held in January. We know he must have been pretty famous in his own time since he pops up in Plato's *Symposium* as a guest alongside other big names Socrates and Alcibiades.

If the surviving works of Aristophanes are anything to go by, Greek comedy was one long *Carry On* movie, if the *Carry On* cast ditched all their knowing looks and double entendres and instead said outright what they meant. Try to imagine this and it'll ruin *Carry On Doctor* for you for life. Nobody needs to see Sid James with an erection when nurse Barbara Windsor does her sexy little wiggly walk through the hospital ward, the explosion of his blood pressure gauge illustrates his emotions perfectly well, thank you. As does a career-best 'Cor' expelled from Bernard Bresslaw with suitably wide eyes. I had never considered *Carry On* films as being an example of the exemplary use of the subtle sex joke before I dived into the works of Aristophanes.

The *Carry On* films' central message that men are all after one thing, the one thing which is never namechecked, is near to the sheer wholesomeness of *The Great British Bake Off* when compared to the opening of Aristophanes' *Lysistrata*. This opening expresses that same sentiment that powered the *Carry On* films but does so openly without the knowing looks, the raised eyebrows, the pinched faces and the 'Oh, Matrons'. 'Tits and clits! Tits and clits! That's what all this is about! That's all they are ever after.'[12]

Aristophanes does not do subtle, the opening scene of his play *The Knights* has two servants masturbating, no doubt making full of use of those leather phalluses sewn into the leotards of the actors.

> Demosthenes: Hehehe, sure is but I'm afraid doing this is going to get me … excoriated! No, no, it won't do; it's a bad omen, this!
>
> Nikias: Excoriated? What are you on about, man?
>
> Demosthenes: Excoriation; it's the wanker's curse, Nikias! Can't do that for ever.[13]

Excoriating means to lose your skin, making this the ancient equivalent of those tales gullible adolescent boys are told by their mates that if you play with it too much it'll fall off/make you go blind.

The Assembly Women, whose plot revolves around what would happen if it were women rather than men who sat in the Athenian assembly, concludes the women would use their newly found powers to legislate on sex. 'The women have hereby decreed that if a man desires to fuck a young woman, he may do so only after he fucks an old one. Further, should this young man refuse to obey by this statute, the older woman shall be authorised to drag the aforesaid young man by his cock, without any legal ramifications to her person or property!'[14]

The young man caught in this situation, Epigenes, finds himself the victim of stage directions such as 'Drops his phallus violently' and 'Young Woman becomes excited and pulls Epigenes by the phallus' and 'Takes his phallus and pulls him in the opposite direction'. This is pure physical comedy.

Penile-style physical comedy is in abundance in *The Thesmophoriazusae*, or *Women at the Festival* in English, whose plot involves Mnesilochus disguising himself as a woman to infiltrate a mass protest by the women of the city. The scene where Mnesilochus' deceit is uncovered by the women particularly stands out.

> Cleisthenes: Stand up straight. What do you keep pushing that thing down for?
>
> First Woman: *peering from behind*
>
> There's no mistaking it.

Cleisthenes: *also peering from behind*

Where has it gone to now?

First Woman: To the front.

Cleisthenes: *from in front*

No.

First Woman: *from behind*

Ah! it's behind now.[15]

You can see here from the dialogue how the stage directions are implied, I'm sure we all have the same sequence running through our heads right now of Mnesilochus popping his faux leather penis back and forth to evade detection. Had ancient Greek theatres possessed roofs, this scene would have brought them tumbling down.

The plot of *The Lysistrata*, in which the women of Greece conspire together to hold a sex strike until a peace deal is signed to end the Peloponnesian Wars, is heavy on erection gags.

[Enter the Spartan Herald. He, too, has a giant erection, which he is trying to hide under his cloak.]

Spartan Herald: Where's the Athenian Senate and the Prytanes? I come with fresh dispatches.

Cinesias [looking at the Herald's erection]: Are you a man, or some phallic monster?

Spartan Herald: I'm a herald, by the twin gods. And my good man, I come from Sparta with a proposal, arrangements for a truce.

Cinesias: If that's the case, why do you have a spear concealed in there?

Spartan Herald: I'm not concealing anything, by god.

Cinesias: Then why are you turning to one side? What's that thing there, sticking from your cloak? Has your journey made your groin inflamed?

Spartan Herald: By old Castor, this man's insane!

Cinesias: You rogue, you've got a hard on!

Spartan Herald: No I don't, I tell you. Let's have no more nonsense.

Cinesias [pointing to the herald's erection]: Then what's that?

Spartan Herald: It's a Spartan herald's stick.[16]

Greek comedy was coarse, it was crude, but it is a vital window into Greek society. Comedy is the antidote to all those philosophers declaring over hundreds of pages their vision for a perfect society and how a true citizen should behave and be, it's the soothing balm of relatability. The ancient Greeks may have been clever fellows producing ideas of such burning brilliance they can spark the inner genius in humankind centuries later, but these titans of intelligence also rubbed at aching ribs, laughing their arses off at an actor waving a leather penis about the stage. The knob gag deserves to be included in that cradle of civilisation, snuggled somewhere between medicine and art, for without it our society would be very different. Would any of us want to live in a world where an amusingly phallic-shaped vegetable did not elicit a smile? Absolutely not.

The stone sausage of man

Earlier in this chapter we looked at the Great Dionysia festival and its procession of supplicants carrying replica phalluses in honour of the god Dionysius. This annual festival was not the only time in ancient Athens where the penis was on full display, it was on full display on every other non-festival day too. Penises could be seen at crossroads, at the borders of land, at the borders of city states, outside temples and the gymnasium and on street corners. Why particularly these places? Because on these spots (and many others besides) there would be placed a Herm.

A Herm was a stone pillar on which was carved a face and an erect penis which jutted out of the middle of the pillar (see Images 39 and 40). Although it is tempting to think of Herms as the product of a lazy, drunk sculptor who, fed up with the perfect proportions of the Doryphoros, went rogue and full-on cubist millennia before cubism was a thing, there was a point to the simplicity of the Herm. It's the same reason why you find Herms at very particular places like on roads and at the edge of fields, the Herm started life as a boundary marker. As the name suggests, Herms were linked to the god Hermes, who amongst his godly roles was helping lost travellers on their journey, a Herm was a certainly a useful marker for the lost and confused. Hermes was also associated with fertility, hence the erect penis acting as an unsubtle representation of this fertility.

Possibly because of their association with travelling, Herms became symbols of luck, luck which could be gained by giving his erect phallus a quick feel. I can say this for a fact because archaeological studies of Herms have shown their phalluses to be shinier than the rest of them. You can see the same effect on the right boob of the statue of Juliet, of *Romeo and Juliet* fame, erected in the courtyard of a house alleged to be hers in Verona, Italy. The boob is shiny gold on an otherwise bronze statue and has been ever since guidebooks started telling tourists it brought good luck. This makes for an interesting afternoon, watching tourists calculate the exact length of time to acquire the promised good luck without looking like some kind of pervert feeling up the likeness of what was a teenage girl.

The crudely shaped, impassively faced, shiny of penis Herms of Athens were to suffer a much greater outrage than the much-photographed molestation of poor Juliet's breast.

The Herm choppers!

The year was 415 BCE and the civil war between the Greek city states known as the Peloponnesian War was now in its seventeenth year. Seventeen years is a long time for any war to be fought, even more so when you remember, Sparta aside, that these were not professional soldiers fighting other professional soldiers but rather armies made up of citizens of the *polis*. During these dark days of a seemingly never-ending war that had dragged into it almost all of Greece, the Athenian assembly was debating on whether to launch an expedition to invade Sicily.

The charismatic and, as we have previously established, drop-dead gorgeous Alcibiades saw invading Sicily as the beginning of a whole new wave of empire for Athens and inspired others to share his dream. 'Many were they who sat in the palaestras and lounging-places mapping out in the sand the shape of Sicily and the position of Libya and Carthage.'[15] Others were distinctly less keen on the idea, chiefly a man named Nicias who tried 'to divert the people from the capture of Syracuse as an undertaking too difficult for them'.[16] So naturally when the assembly voted for the invasion they gave the generalship of the whole expedition to Alcibiades and Nicias. There is something to be said for making those who shout the loudest for war experience it firsthand, but it seems jolly unfair to poor Nicias, who found himself elected general of an expedition he'd been arguing was doomed 'against his will'.[17]

As the Athenian fleet prepared to set sail for an expedition one of the generals in charge of it was convinced would fail, it is fair to say the atmosphere in the city was edgy. So edgy that an astrologer named Meton went mad and burnt down his own house to get his son excused from being part of the Sicilian invasion on compassionate grounds. Which you would have thought might have given Alcibiades a moment's pause, or a smidgen of pondering to wonder what hell of a future Meton had foreseen in the stars that had propelled him to such a drastic action. It didn't because Alcibiades was not a man who thought beyond the immediate moment he was in, which is why his life was as interesting as it was. Alcibiades' life was less a rollercoaster and more of a log flume that wound him to the pinnacle of success before a steep plunge down accompanied by an enormous eruption of water that left him and all those in his near vicinity soaked to the skin and shivering. The Sicily expedition was the top of the log flume as far as Alcibiades could see and he was ready, wired and willing for the ascent, Nicias held fast beside him underneath the metal bar when something happened that really did make the Athenians stop and think.

One morning, the city awoke to find a heinous crime had been committed. 'All the stone Hermae in the city of Athens, that is to say the customary square figures, so common in the doorways of private houses and temples, had in one night most of them their faces mutilated.'[18] The Herm Choppers had struck!

Herms being considered symbols of good luck and linked specifically to travel, this dreadful act was 'thought to be ominous for the expedition'.[19] Suspicion initially fell on rival city state, Corinth, who possessed the motivation for attempting to intimidate Athens into abandoning their expedition, for Corinth had founded several colonies on Sicily that were now under threat. However, annoyingly there didn't appear to be any evidence that Corinthian agents had sneaked into the city en masse during the night armed with mallets, chisels and other toolbox must-haves and beaten the Herms of the city to a distressingly crumbling state.

Who else besides the Corinthians might want to frighten the city into abandoning the military operation they had been so keen to vote for? Which was when suspicions were turned inwards towards those Athenians who had been vocally against the Sicilian expedition; had they really graciously accepted the vote that had gone against their beliefs or were they playing the role that they had, whilst secretly seeking a way to subvert the democratic vote? Were they looking to subvert democracy entirely? There was a distinct possibility they might have been, democracy as a political system was not popular with political thinkers, who feared the tyranny of the many (possibly this now included Nicias, who'd been appointed to a position he never sought and certainly didn't want by a democratic vote) and fears began to spread that a revolution was in the making. Something had to be done.

'Large public rewards were offered to find the authors; and it was further voted that anyone who knew of any other act of impiety having been committed should come and give information without fear of consequences, whether he were citizen, alien, or slave.'[18] Money is a great incentive and informants scuttered forwards to dish out tales to the authorities. However, these tales that the informants were so eager to divulge were not foreign agents nor internal dissenters but rather they brought stories of 'some previous mutilations of other images perpetrated by young men in drunken frolic'.[19]

Now this sounds about right and as neat a solution as can be found – a load of pissed-up youngsters post-*symposium* found something that amused them, the sort of thing that entertains the inebriated only. No sober person has ever thought pissing into a wishing well a worthwhile thing to do, nor found hilarity posting individual chips from a late-night fish-and-chip supper through the letterboxes of an entire street of houses, nor picking up a random traffic cone from the road and taking it home with them. Into this camp of things you think will make the hangover worth it but won't we can add smashing in the faces and other bits of those silly old Herms; it was all a bit of hermless fun (typo intended because that is an epically good pun and it needs to be heard).

'The multitude, however, were not moved by this reasoning, nor by that of those who thought the affair no terrible sign at all, but rather one of the common effects of strong wine, when dissolute youth, in mere sport, are carried away into wanton acts. They looked on the occurrence with wrath and fear.'[20] This multitude could not be persuaded this was hermless fun (it's too good a pun not to use it again), they needed it to be more, and in such an atmosphere of wrath and fear villains had to be found.

Under public pressure the authorities were forced to act, 'the council and the assembly convening for this purpose many times within a few days'.[21] Androcles proved very helpful to the assembly by producing a gang of eyewitnesses who could all positively identify the guilty parties, true, those eyewitnesses are described as being aliens and slaves, so not good, decent citizens whose word could be trusted. Also true, the guilty party they finger was Alcibiades, which makes absolutely no sense if this were a conspiracy rather than drunken shenanigans. Why would Alcibiades want to make the expedition he was so keen to lead look inauspicious? On the other hand, I can quite believe Alcibiades and chums mutilated the Herms whilst off their tits on wine and feeling overly exuberant about the forthcoming Sicilian jaunt.

Alcibiades protested his innocence, but suggested they sort the whole thing out when he got back from successfully conquering Sicily. Which he didn't, because hearing of Androcles ramping things up in Athens whilst he was off playing the general, Alcibiades did a runner, threw himself on the mercy of the Spartan enemies and was condemned by his home city in his absence. This could well be an indicator that it was indeed Alcibiades who was the instigator of the Herm chopping, it could be a sign that not long into his Sicilian expedition he realised Nicias had been correct the whole time and that he was not going to return home as an all-conquering general who could sweep aside such petty accusations as criminal damage and upsetting the all-powerful and malevolently menacing gods. Or it could be that Alcibiades simply panicked for this own life and threw himself on the mercy of the enemy because he didn't know what else to do.

And no, in case you are wondering, Sicily was not conquered. It was an utter defeat for Athens, a devastating one that wiped out a sizeable proportion of the Athenian fleet to the extent that some historians believe that this was the tipping point of the entire Peloponnesian War. That would be the

Peloponnesian War that Sparta won, occupying the crushed Athens and abolished history's first-ever democracy, replacing it with a tyranny. And all because some drunken youths thought it would be funny to mess about with those stone pillars with jutting knobs!

Lucky dicks

You don't mess with the penis, no, you utilise it because it's vibrating with good luck. This lucky nature of the penis/phallus and its ability to ward off bad luck/evil is why it is quite so ubiquitous in ancient Greece. You will find phallus-shaped jewellery, phallus friezes, phallus windchimes and images of phalluses splashed across crockery.

So common was the phallic image that it was rendered innocuous and everyday to the ancient Greeks. The same cannot be said for the twenty-first century, which is why we find such images shocking, grotesque and even offensive. You will never see an erect penis on British TV, for example. Nor will you see anyone, outside of some very dubious nightclubs/social gatherings involving a bowl of car keys, wearing a penis necklace and I feel confident stating that the wooden door of your local village church is not flanked by statues of ten-foot-tall penises. This, undoubtedly, is the reason why the weather in Britain is one long streak of grey mizzle; lucky penises are needed.

Part III

Women

Chapter 9

A Punishment from the Gods

Let us recap, so far we've covered the body beautiful (of men), sport (for men), love affairs (between men), wild dinner parties (for men) and the abundance of images of genitalia (belonging to men). The question begs to be asked: where are all the women?

Let us start from the beginning with the very first woman; her name was Pandora, and she did not have a box. What Pandora did have was a jar, that due to a translation error along the centuries became a box, but more on that jar later.

Origin myths for humankind are something that all the major religions cover. In the Judaeo-Christian tradition, God pencilled the creation of men and women on day six of what had been a very busy week for him. Having created the earth, the heavens, light, darkness, water, trees, fish, birds and all other animals on his to do list, God then made mankind.

> So God created mankind in his own image,
> in the image of God he created them;
> male and female he created them.
>
> God blessed them and said to them, 'Be fruitful and increase in number; fill the earth and subdue it. Rule over the fish in the sea and the birds in the sky and over every living creature that moves on the ground.'[1]

With all the satisfaction of someone who has successfully put together an IKEA bookcase without a single leftover screw, 'God saw all that he had made, and it was very good.'[2] So much so that he allows himself to put down that Allen key and rest on day seven before he'll even consider putting together those bunkbeds. In Hinduism, Brahma the Creator out of loneliness split himself in two: male and female. In the Islamic text the Qur'an, Allah moulds man from clay, 'and breathed into him My spirit'.[3]

What all these explanations for the existence of men and women have in common is good intentions and acting as a reflection of their creator. Yes, I'm aware that Adam and Eve are about to imminently screw it all up and mankind has hardly covered itself in glory and done God proud, sorry, God. But humans, both men and women, were created in a spirit of positivity we can say even if we haven't lived up to those creator's expectations, sorry again, God. In Greek mythology, Pandora, the first woman, was created as a punishment.

The crime for which Pandora was the penalty had been committed by the Titan, Prometheus. In Greek mythology, Titans were the deities who governed the heavens and earth under the leadership of Kronos, until they were replaced by the Olympian gods led by Kronos' son, Zeus. If you suspect there's a hell of a backstory about why Zeus turned against his father so viciously and stole his crown, you are entirely correct. It's a revenge story laden with family dynamics and hatred that no Hollywood film has ever come close to bettering, probably because it involves cannibalism and castration, two themes that are not known crowd pleasers (although both would considerably improve whatever superhero movie is coming out next).

Zeus may have turned on his own father during the Titans-versus-Olympians war of the gods, but he was not alone in being a turncoat, or rather a turn-chiton; Prometheus was a Titan who fought for the Olympian gods. This really should not have come as a surprise to anyone given that Prometheus was the god of forethought, crafty counsel and trickery. Prometheus had 'not to be trusted' pretty much tattooed across his forehead. What is surprising, given the ease of his treachery to the Titans, is that the newly enthroned head god, Zeus, should entrust Prometheus with the very important job of moulding mankind out of clay and somehow not foresee that the god of crafty trickery was unlikely to follow the strict instructions he'd been left.

The instruction pertinent to our tale that Prometheus was given, and paid no attention to, was that mankind was not to know the secret of how to make fire. If you're wondering why Zeus didn't want mankind to have access to fire it's because Greek gods are mean and delight in mucking around with the lives of mortal men to make them more difficult than they need to be. 'For the gods keep hidden the means of life. Else you would easily do work enough in a day to supply you for a whole year.'[4] This is why the gods need venerating and sacrificing to, not because they are worthy of honours and deserve such veneration for some noble action performed, but rather to stop them being even meaner to you.

Not best pleased with Prometheus breaking the god code by bestowing upon mankind the means to make buttered toast, Zeus came up with the perfect response: 'But I will give men as the price for fire an evil thing in which they may all be glad of heart whilst they embrace their own destruction, So said the father of men and gods and laughed aloud.'[5] This is a phrase you will find often in this book as a reminder and because it cannot be stressed often enough, Greek gods are nothing like the Christian god. During the tale of Pandora, you will see Zeus as less of a god, from what we understand a god to be, and more of a supervillain, complete with his own team of henchmen and henchwomen who will guffaw on cue.

Zeus assembled a crack team from amongst his Olympian henchmen and women to construct the perfect vengeance. Hephaestus, the god of artisans, created the exterior of this punishment for mankind, it was: 'a sweet, lovely maiden shape'.[6] Athena, the goddess of wisdom, taught this newly created maiden needlework; Aphrodite, goddess of love, gave her 'cruel longing and cares that weary the limbs';[7] and the messenger god Hermes' contribution was 'a shameless mind and a deceitful nature'.[8] Their creation was then dressed real pretty and sent to live amongst men, who at that time were, 'free from ills and hard toil and heavy sickness',[9] as a ticking time bomb programmed to obliterate their comfortable world.

The punishment mankind was to have inflicted upon it sounds awful until you hear what Zeus inflicted upon Prometheus as his penance: the Titan was tethered to a rock and an eagle sent down to peck out his liver. Which doesn't sound much fun, but it gets even worse because each night Prometheus' liver would regenerate itself so that come morning that same eagle could fly down and peck it out all over again. Yikes!

Pandora's incendiary device was a jar and when she thoughtlessly uncorked it she released sickness and toil, along with sorrow and mischief upon men. Thus bringing to an end a golden era for mankind to which they could never return. Whoops. However, left in the jar, after all the evils that hurt mankind had poofed out the windows, was hope. It had got stuck under the rim.

To be fair to Pandora, in all the myths we have about her, nowhere does anyone tell her not to open that jar. Which perhaps reveals something about the psyche of Greek men, they really don't like having their stuff messed about with. The Pandora myth is also very revealing on how women were thought of in Greek society, she is sent as a punishment for men and her actions make their lives considerably worse. This is not me viewing Pandora through some twenty-first-century feminist lens, inferring a meaning from a tale that isn't there about ancient Greek men's deep distrust and suspicion of women. I don't need to infer anything or search for hints behind words, because here are the words.

'From her is the race of women and female kind; of her is the deadly race and tribe of women who live amongst mortal men to their great trouble, no helpmates in hateful poverty but only in wealth,'[10] says eighth-century BCE poet Hesiod, not so much as nailing his colours to the wall but also to the trees, bushes and any passing squirrels. He follows this statement on the nature of women with a bee analogy so precise that one can almost picture him staring at a hive in silent, fuming rage, jaw clenched. 'Throughout the day until the sun goes down the bees are busy and lay their white combs, while the drones stay at home in the covered skeps and reap the toil of others into their own bellies.'[11]

There is a similarly so-weirdly-specific-it-must-be-based-on-his-own-life line in Hesiod's poem *Works and Days*: 'Do not let a flaunting woman coax and cozen and deceive you; she is after your barn. The man who trusts womankind trusts deceivers.'[12] Presumably composed as he stared at his lost barn in silent, fuming rage, jaw clenched. Remember the attributes that the messenger god Hermes bestowed upon Pandora – 'a deceitful nature' was one of them. Hesiod sees this reflected in the women of his time.

Also of Hesiod's time, the eighth/seventh centuries BCE, was a poet by the name of Semonides who lived on the island of Armogos, a tiny speck of a land whose population in 2011 was only numbered at 1,973 people. Unlike with Hesiod, whose two works *Theogony* and *Works and Days* have made it to the twenty-first century intact, we have only fragments of most of Semonides' poetry. The only full poem by Semonides that has survived is called *The Nature of Women* and possesses the unique power of making you grateful that the rest of his output has been lost. A sentiment clearly felt by whoever contributed to the Wikipedia entry on *The Nature of Women*: 'Despite the poem's length and its interest as evidence as to early Greek attitudes towards women, it has received little scholarly attention and has generally been considered to be of little literary merit.'[13] Bitchy.

The Nature of Women is one big, long rant about how awful women expressed by comparing them to various animals. If you want a feel for just how unpleasant a poem this is, here is the opening line. 'From the start the Gods made women different. One type is from a pig – a hairy sow whose house is a rolling heap of filth, and she herself unbathed in unwashed clothes, reposes on the shit pile growing fat.'[14]

Elsewhere the women derived from a dog is a 'no good bitch'. 'No man can shut her up with threats, not even if in the grip of anger he smashes her teeth with a rock, nor even by speaking in a sweet manner, even if by chance she is sitting among guests she will keep on barking and nothing can stop her.'[15]

And so it goes on, the fox woman is devious, the grey ass woman is used 'to get smacked and won't give in until you really force her',[16] the weasel woman is sex crazed and a thief, the horse woman is lazy, the ape woman is ugly and a laughing stock. The only woman worth anything in Semonides' world is the bee woman. 'Zeus gratifies mankind with these most excellent and thoughtful wives,'[17] he says and then adds, 'All these other types are here to stay side by side with man forever. Yes, Zeus made this greatest pain of all; Woman.'[18]

We shall now pause for an interlude where all the female readers of this book collectively decide that Semonides is a slug and they'd all like to be the foot that squishes him into the patio, even if he is attempting to be funny.

Hesiod and Semonides may have settled on all of womankind to suffer the stabs of their pen, but another seventh-century BCE Greek poet used his barbed words for a more pointed and personal attack. The poet's name was Archilochus and he resided on the island of Paros between the years 680 and 645 BCE. Archilochus had found his woman, Neobule, and was ready to settle down and get going with the whole marriage thing when his betrothed's father, Lycambes, decided on reflection he'd much rather his daughter married someone else.

Marriages being a deal brokered between families, Lycambes' abrupt change of mind was shaming, it showed him to be a man who could not be trusted on his word. It also showed him to be a man unfamiliar with poets and the nasty streak of bitterness that taints their verses.

Paros is a small island, only 75 square miles in size, you can drive right round it in an hour. On such a small island it is highly likely that everyone knew everyone else and their business, Archilochus' broken engagement had to be a talking point, and if it hadn't had been Archilochus was about to make it so. Archilochus was not the sort of man who dealt with a bruised ego and broken heart by smiling in public, acting as if it didn't bother him in the slightest, and then bursting into tears the moment he shut his front door. He was not the type of man to spend his evenings banging his head on the kitchen table and sobbing over his broken engagement. No, Archilochus was the type of man whose hurt feelings festered inside him like the contents of a forgotten fruit bowl, spotting with mould and decaying into a mushy black pulp.

The mushy black pulp inside Archilochus was exorcised by the sweeping of pen across papyri. Unlike Hesiod's unnamed barn-stealing hussy, Archilochus' poem names his ex-fiancée, Neobule, and makes it very clear how he feels about her; it reads like the ancient equivalent of revenge porn.

> Neobule I have forgotten, believe me, do.
> Any man who wants her may have her.
> Aiai! She's past her day, ripening rotten.
> The petals of her flower are all brown.
> The grace that first she had is shot.
> Don't you agree that she looks like a boy?
> A woman like that would drive a man crazy.
> She should get herself a job as a scarecrow.
> I'd as soon hump her as [kiss a goat's butt].[19]

Archilochus' attempts to wound and enact his revenge upon those who had humiliated him worked a little too well; it is said that Lycambes, Neobule and possibly some of her sisters all committed suicide after reading the poem. Which is quite something, if true. Archilochus' pen had power

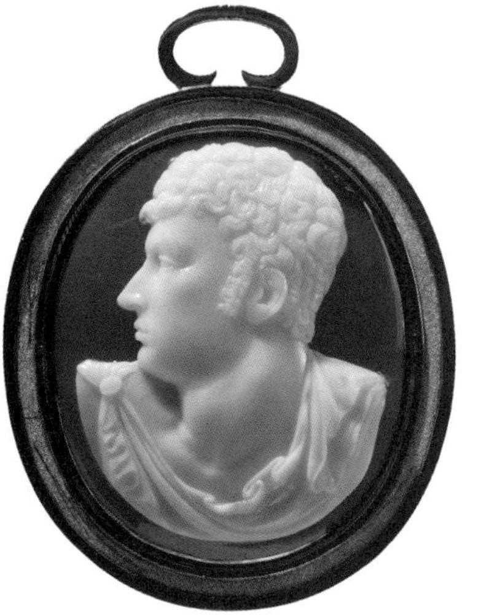

1. Cameo of Lord Byron, an ancient Greece fanboy. (Cameo of Lord George Gordon Byron, The Milton Weil Collection, 1940, Metropolitan Museum of Art, New York, USA)

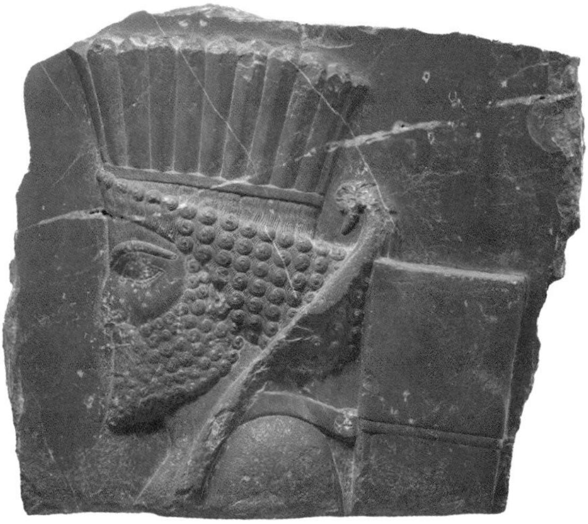

2. A Persian Guard, an example of the 'otherness' that inspired a new notion of being Greek. (Head of a Persian Guard, Purchase, Joseph Pulitzer Bequest, 1955, Metropolitan Museum of Art, New York, USA)

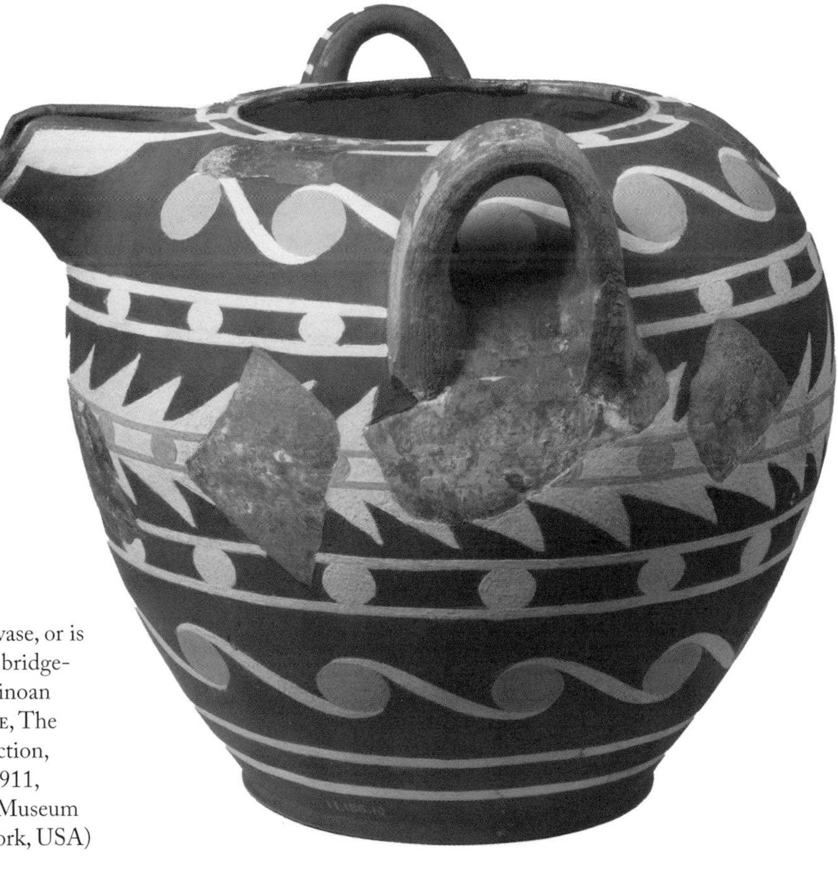

3. A Minoan vase, or is it? (Terracotta bridge-spouted jar, Minoan 1900–1600 BCE, The Cesnola Collection, by exchange, 1911, Metropolitan Museum of Art, New York, USA)

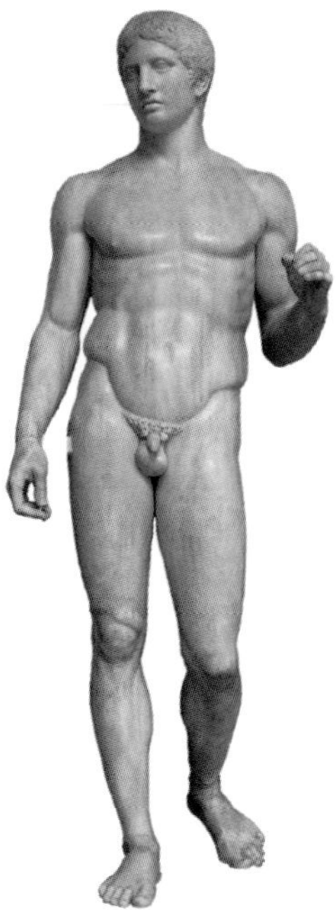

4. The perfect man? A copy of the gorgeous Doryphoros by Polykleitos. (Doryphoros, Credit: Marie-Lan Ngyuen, image and Paolo Villa, backbround, Wikmedia Commons)

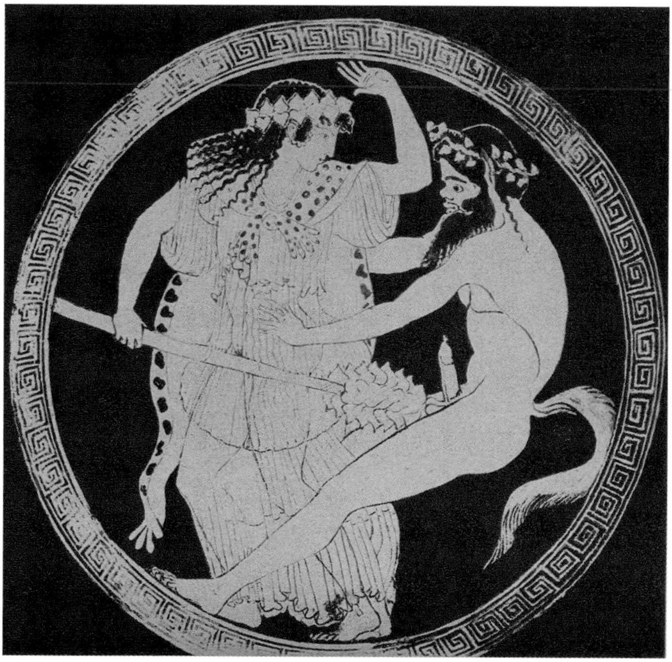

5. A satyr tries it on with a nymph. (A depiction of a Maenad holding a thyrsus aimed at the erect penis of a seated satyr. Colour process print, 1921. Wellcome Collection)

6. A man and his horse hang out in the nude together. (Terracotta cup featuring a horse and groom. Gift of Norbert Schimmel Trust, 1989, Metropolitan Museum of Art, New York, USA)

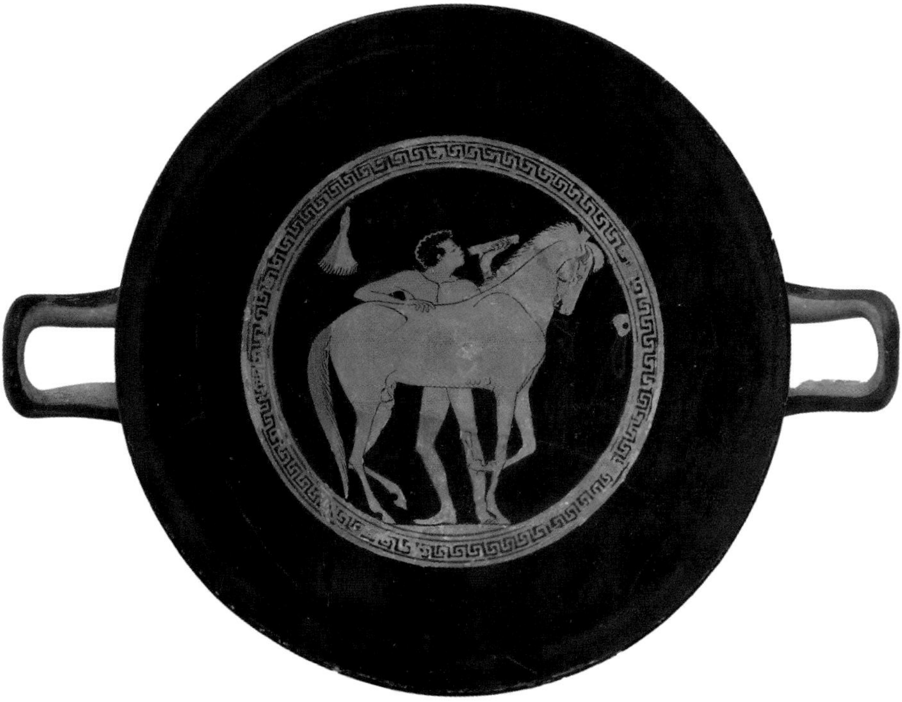

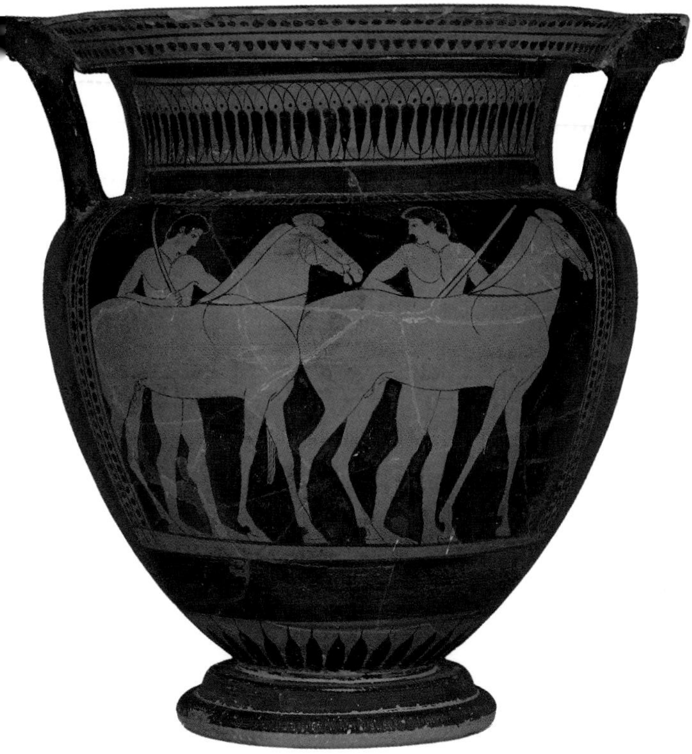

7. Two young lads go riding together. (Two men and horse, Attic Red-Figure Column Krater, attributed to Myson (Greek (Attic), active 500–475 BC), Getty Open Access)

. A young man is torn between work and play, the javelin or the pickaxe. (Youth with thletic equipment. Attic Red-Figure Cup Type B, attributed to the Brygos Painter Greek (Attic), active about 490–470 BC], Getty Open Access)

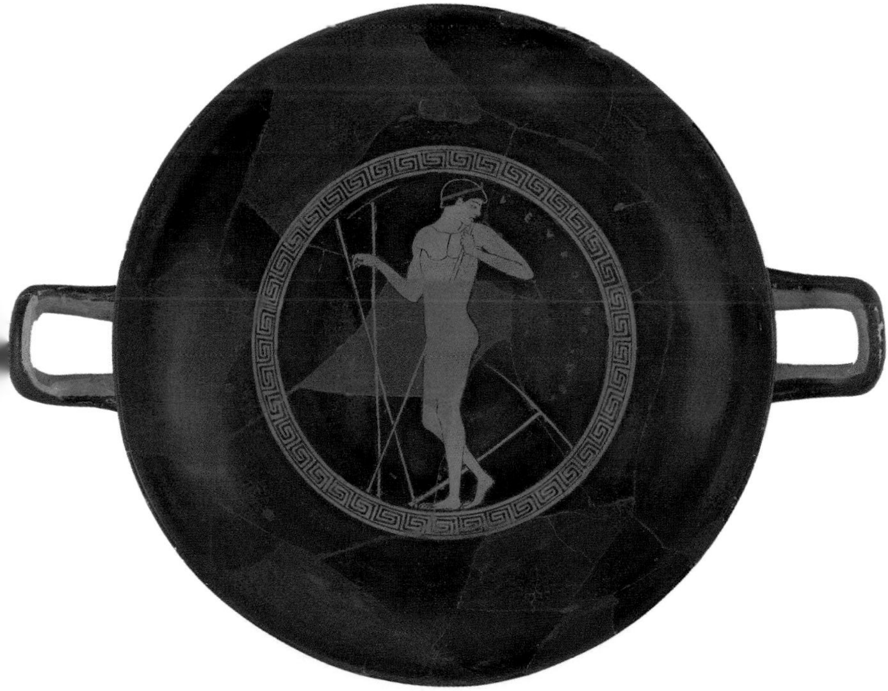

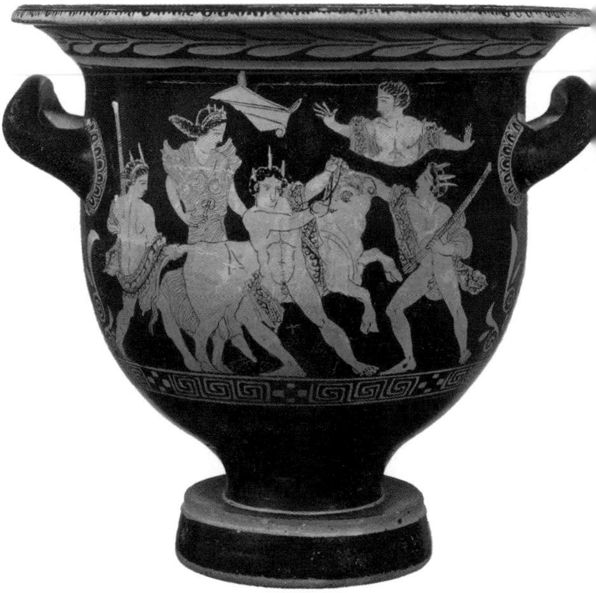

9. Sacrificial ceremony being performed. (Sacrificial Scene. Terracotta bell-krater Fletcher Fund, 1956, Metropolitan Museum of Art, New York, USA)

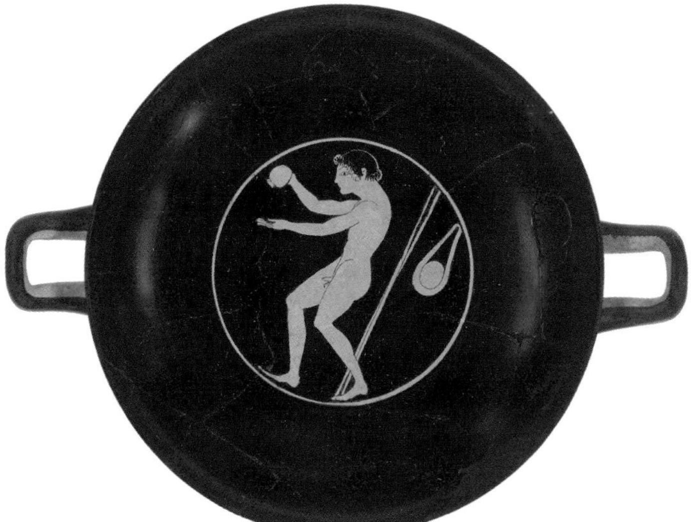

10. A Greek athlete oils up. (Greek athlete with oil. Attic Red-Figure Cup Type C, Attributed to the Ambrosios Painter [Greek (Attic), active 510–500 BC] Getty Open Access)

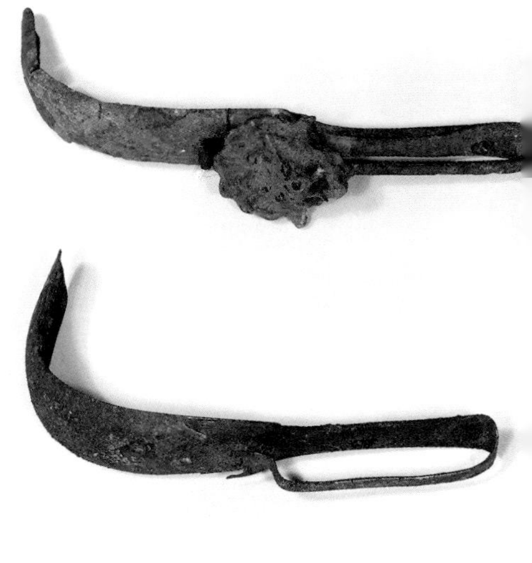

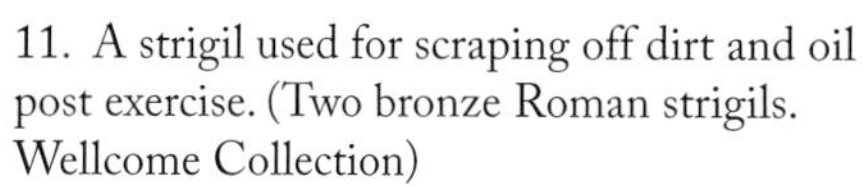

11. A strigil used for scraping off dirt and oil post exercise. (Two bronze Roman strigils. Wellcome Collection)

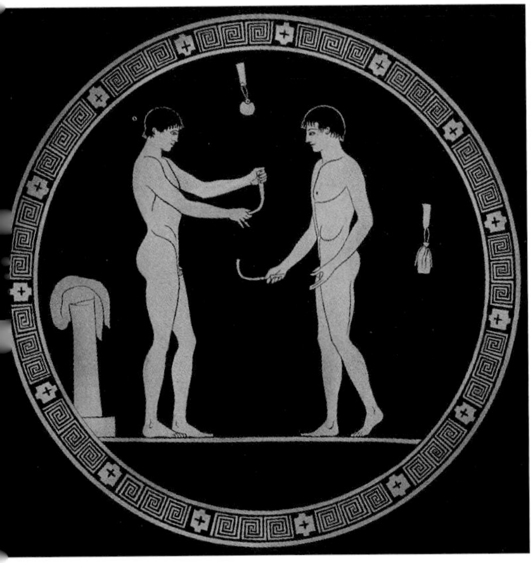

12. Two athletes ready to strigil each other's backs. (Two young men using strigils. Gouache painting by S. W. Kelly, 1937. Wellcome Collection)

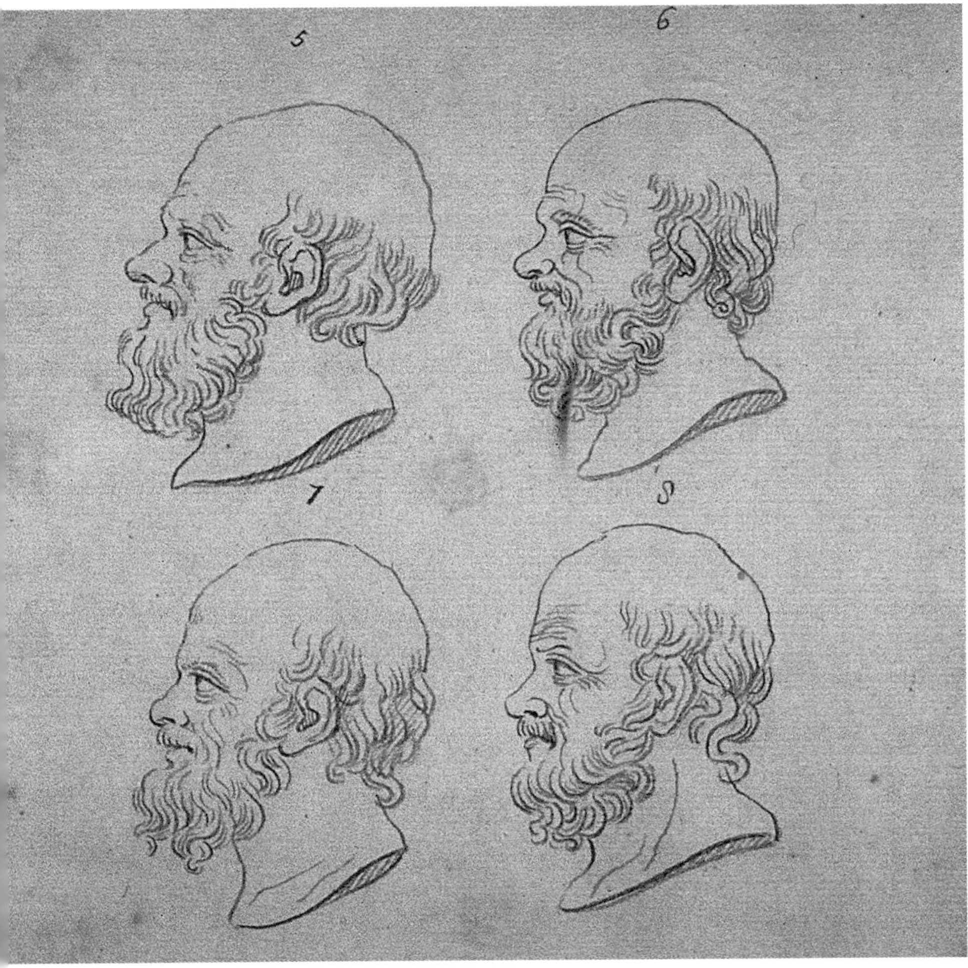

13. Portraits of Socrates. (Likenesses of Socrates, c. 1789. Wellcome Collection)

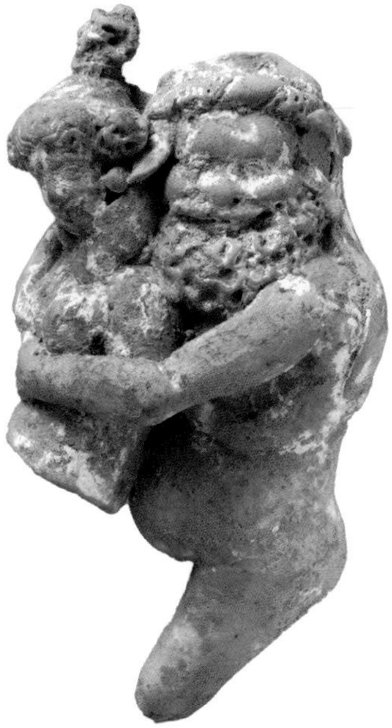

14. A Socratic-looking satyr. (Terracotta statuette of a Satyr and maenad, Rogers Fund 1909, Metropolitan Museum of Art, New York, USA)

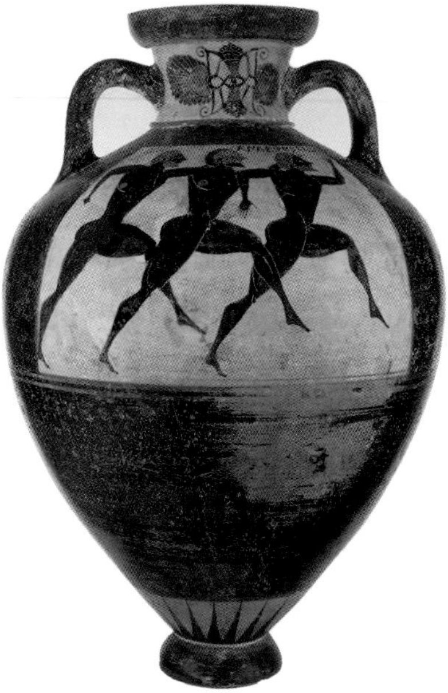

15. From the sixth century, victors at the Panhellenic Games wer awarded a jar filled with olive oil. The image shows the event they won, in this case clearly a running race. (A Running Race. Terracotta Panathenaic prize amphora [jar], The Bothmer Purch Fund, 1978, Metropolitan Museum of Art, New York, USA)

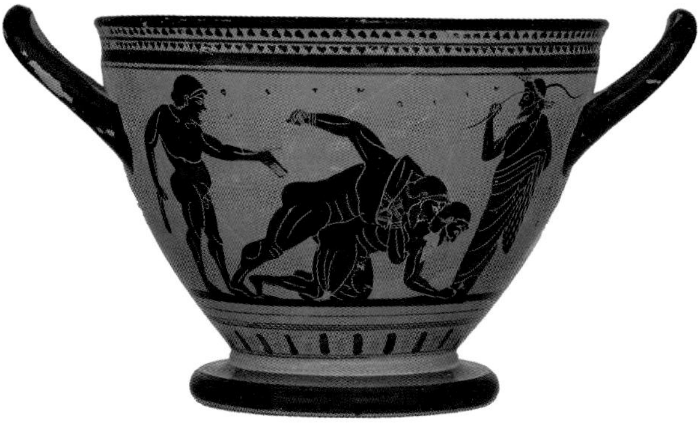

16. The pankration depicted on a drinking cup. Note the judges either side, one holds a whip and the other something that greatly resembles a cosh/truncheon. (A Pankration Competition, Terracotta skyphos [deep drinking cup], Rogers Fund 1906, Metropolitan Museum of Art, New York, US.)

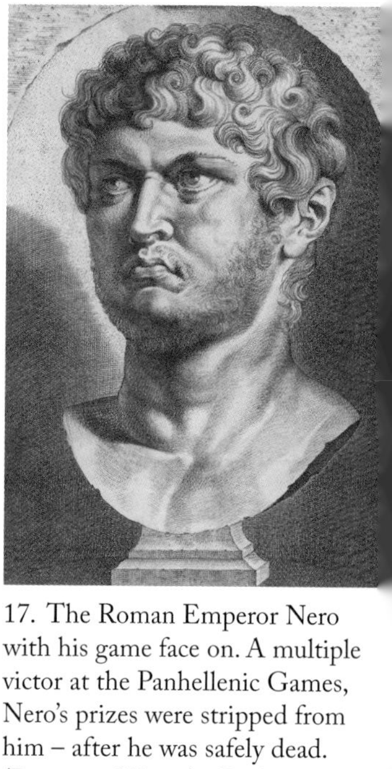

17. The Roman Emperor Nero with his game face on. A multiple victor at the Panhellenic Games, Nero's prizes were stripped from him – after he was safely dead. (Portrait of Nero by Paulus Pontius Bequest of Phyllis Massar 2011, Metropolitan Museum of Art, New York, USA)

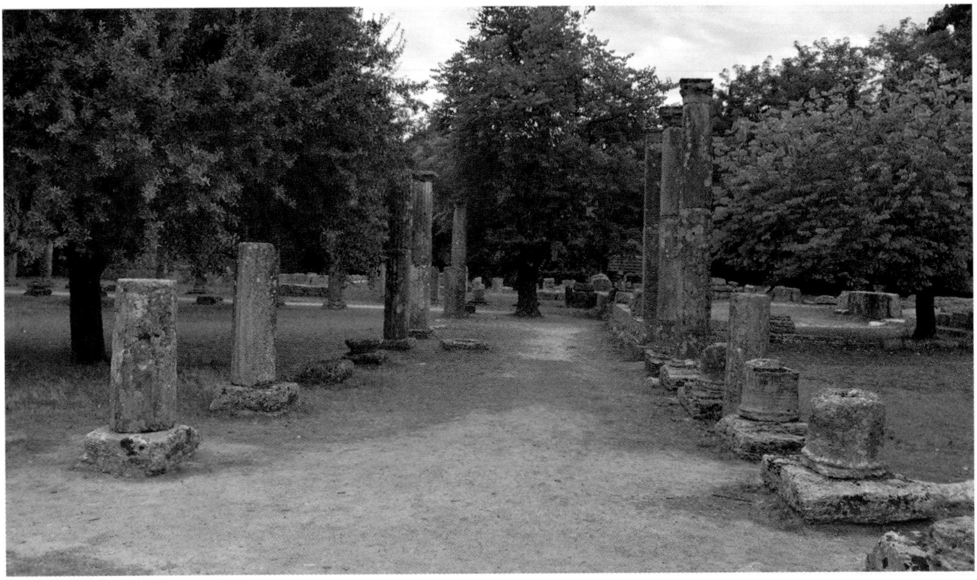

18. Some of what remains of the majestic site of ancient Olympia. (Archaeological site of Ancient Olympia, credited to Annatsach, Wikimedia Commons)

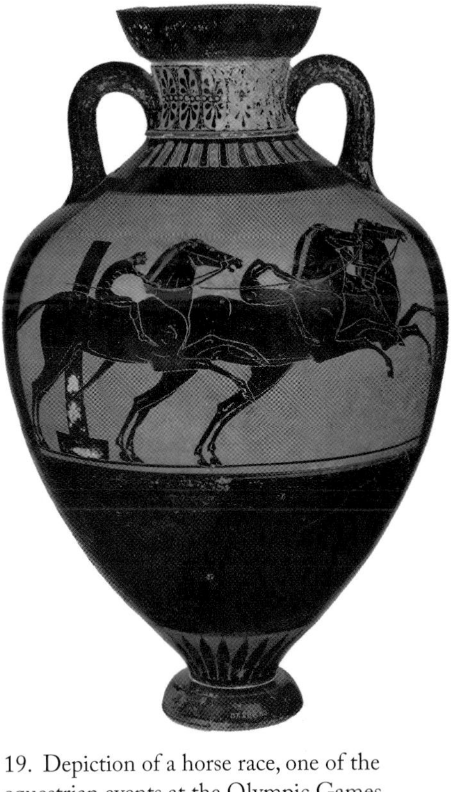

19. Depiction of a horse race, one of the equestrian events at the Olympic Games. (A horse race. Terracotta Panathenaic prize amphora [jar], Rogers Fund 1904, Metropolitan Museum of Art, New York, USA)

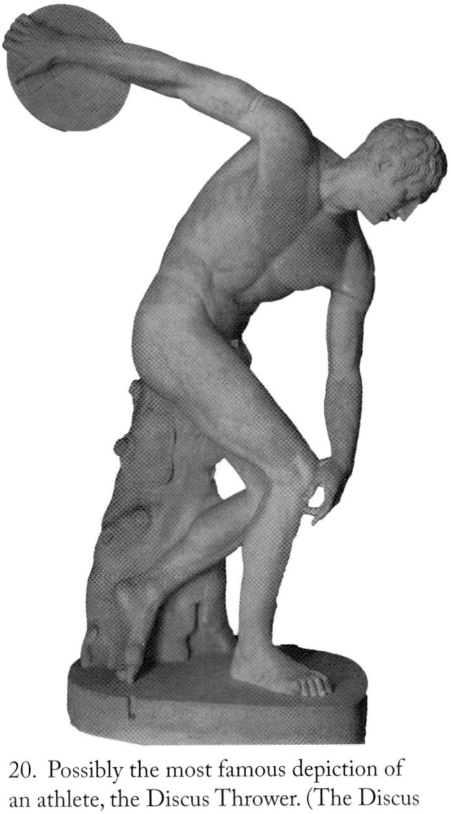

20. Possibly the most famous depiction of an athlete, the Discus Thrower. (The Discus Thrower, Roma, Vaticano, Discobolo di Mirone, Getty Open Access)

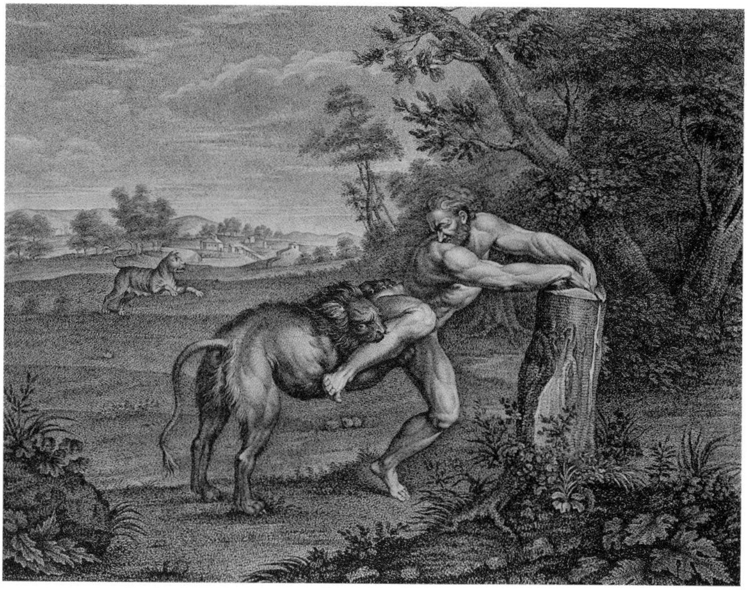

21. The mega famous athlete Milo of Croton who died in a bizarre tree accident depicted here. (Milo of Croton. Woodcut by N. Boldrini after G. A. Pordenone. Wellcome Collection)

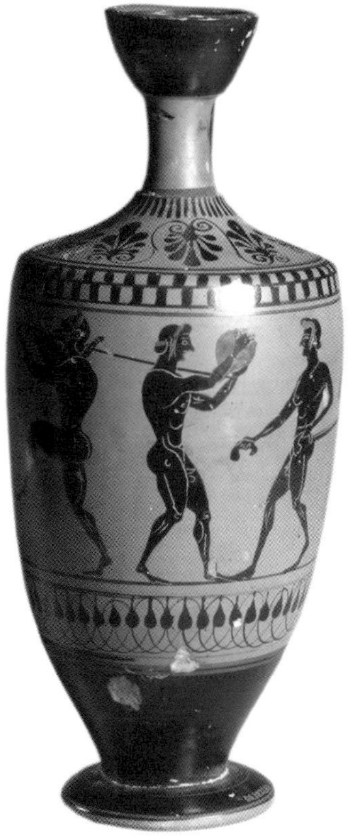

22. Greek Athletes letting it all hang out in the gym. (Athletes practising. Terracotta lekythos (oil flask), Rogers Fund, 1906, Metropolitan Museum of Art, New York, USA)

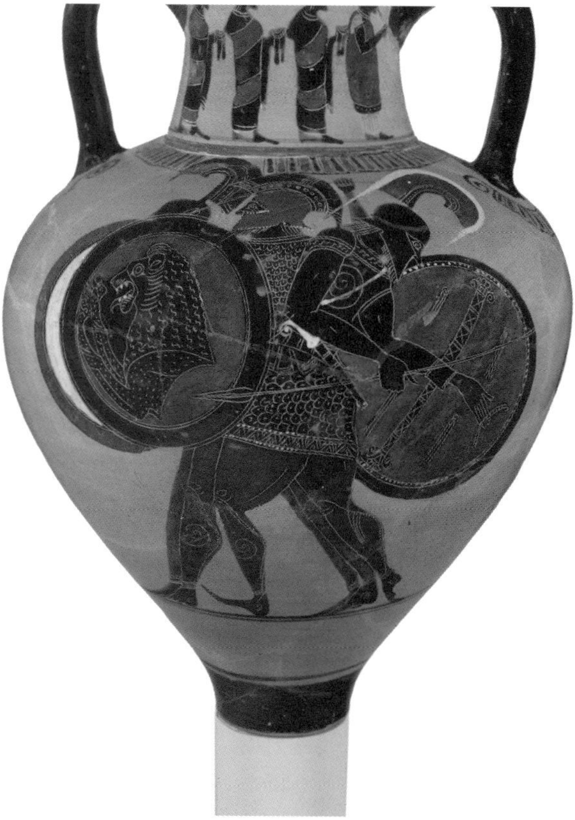

23. Hoplite soldiers, note the massiveness of the shields. Not easy to run with. (Hoplite soldiers, Terracotta neck-amphora (jar), The Bothmer Purchase Fund, 2010, Metropolitan Museum of Art, New York, USA)

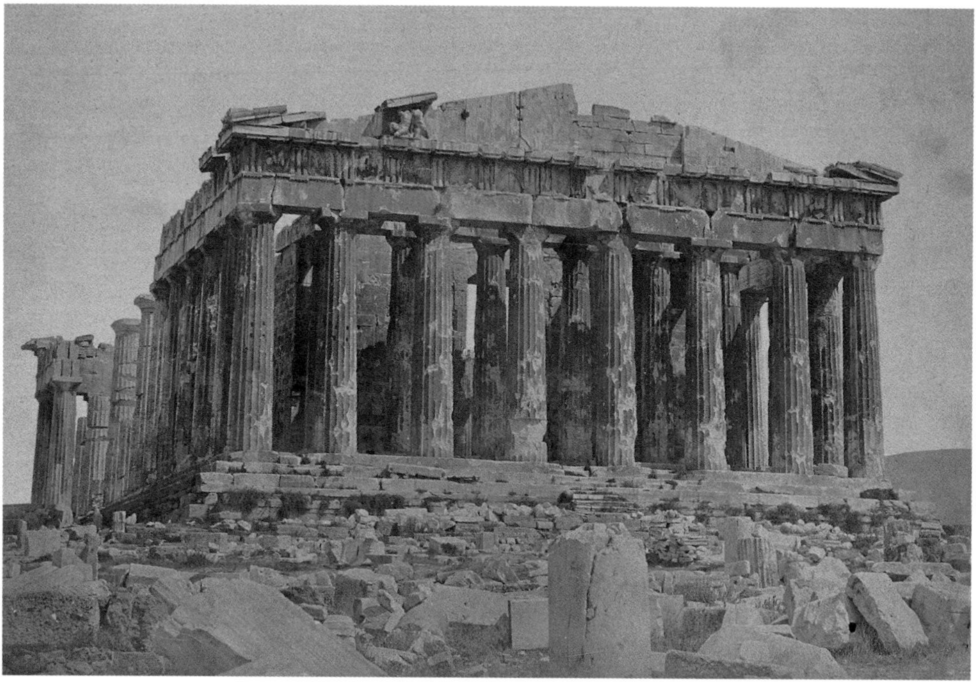

24. The Parthenon in Athens, a physical reminder of their victory over the Persians. (The Parthenon, Greece. Photograph [by Petros Moraites?], ca. 1870. Wellcome Collection)

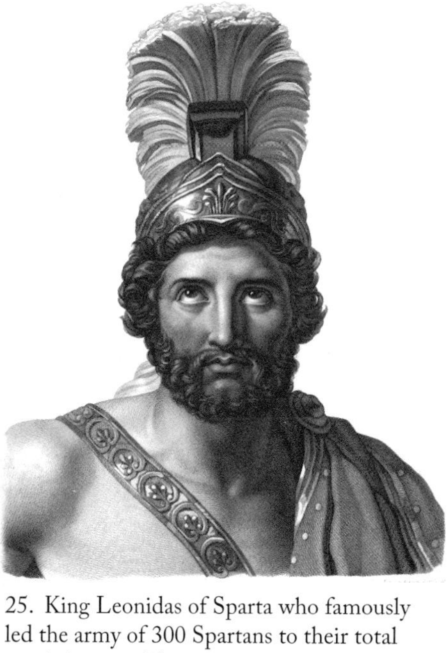

25. King Leonidas of Sparta who famously led the army of 300 Spartans to their total annihilation at Thermopylae to buy time for the rest of Greece to mobilise against the Persians. (Leonidas at Thermopylae. Crayon manner print by N. Bertrand, 1821, after Laguiche after J. L. David, Wellcome Collection)

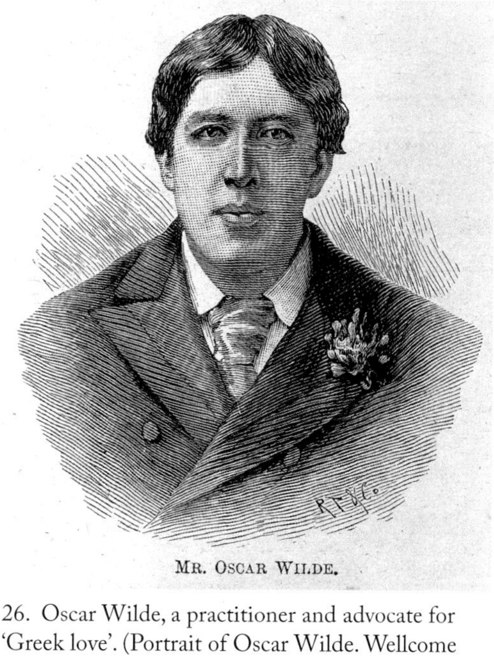

26. Oscar Wilde, a practitioner and advocate for 'Greek love'. (Portrait of Oscar Wilde. Wellcome Collection)

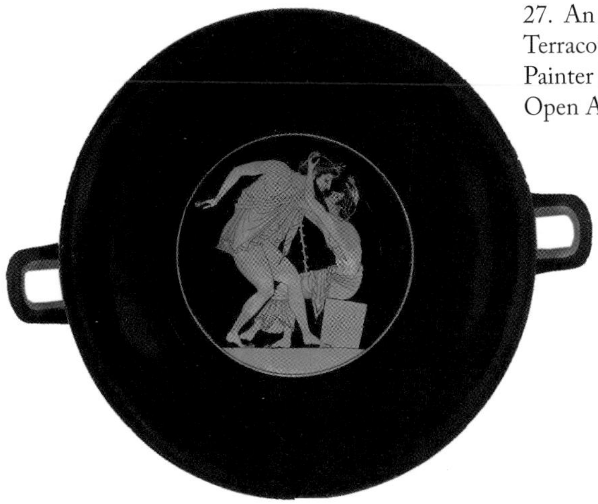

27. An *erastes* and his *eromenos*. (Man with Youth. Terracotta drinking cup, attributed to Carpenter Painter [Greek (Attic), active 515–500 BC], Getty Open Access.)

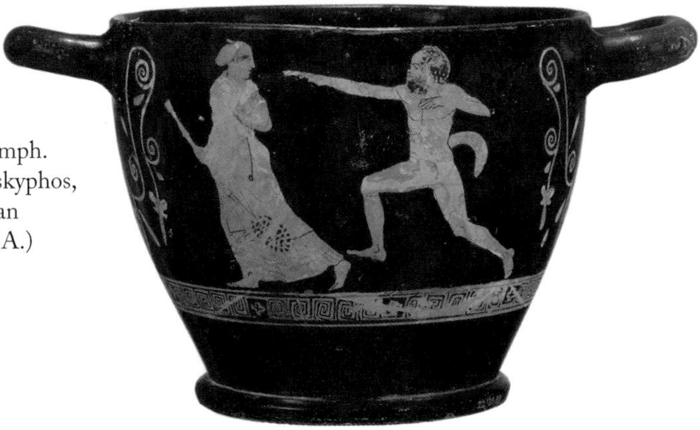

28. A horny satyr pursues a nymph. (Nymph and Satyr. Terracotta skyphos, Rogers Fund 1922, Metropolitan Museum of Art, New York, USA.)

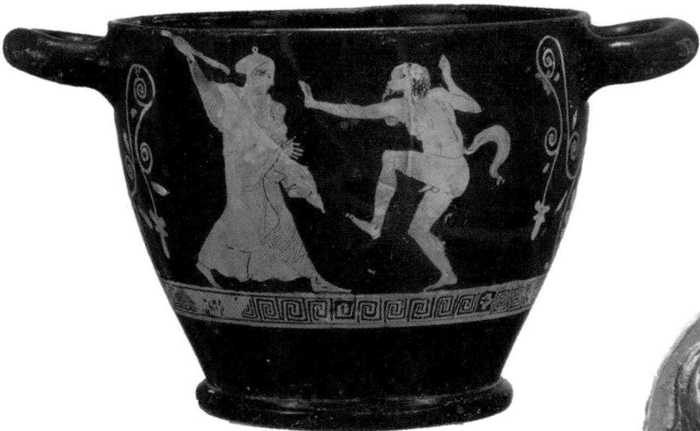

29. An enraged nymph goes on the attack against a horny satyr. (Nymph and Satyr. Terracotta skyphos, Rogers Fund 1922, Metropolitan Museum of Art, New York, USA.)

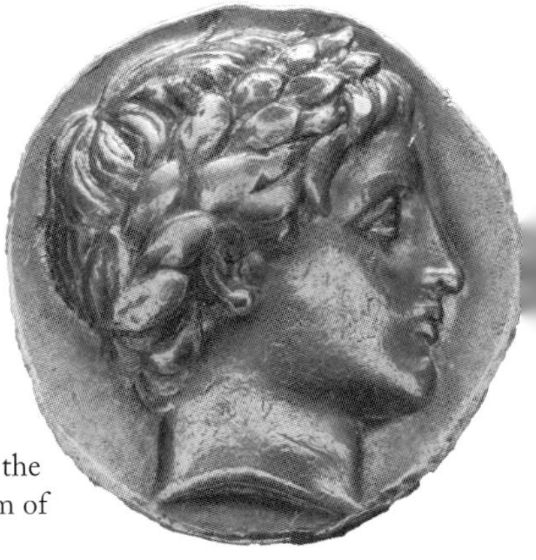

30. Alexander the Great, gay or not? (Gold coin of Alexander the Great, Gift of J. Pierpont Morgan 1905, Metropolitan Museum of Art, New York, USA.)

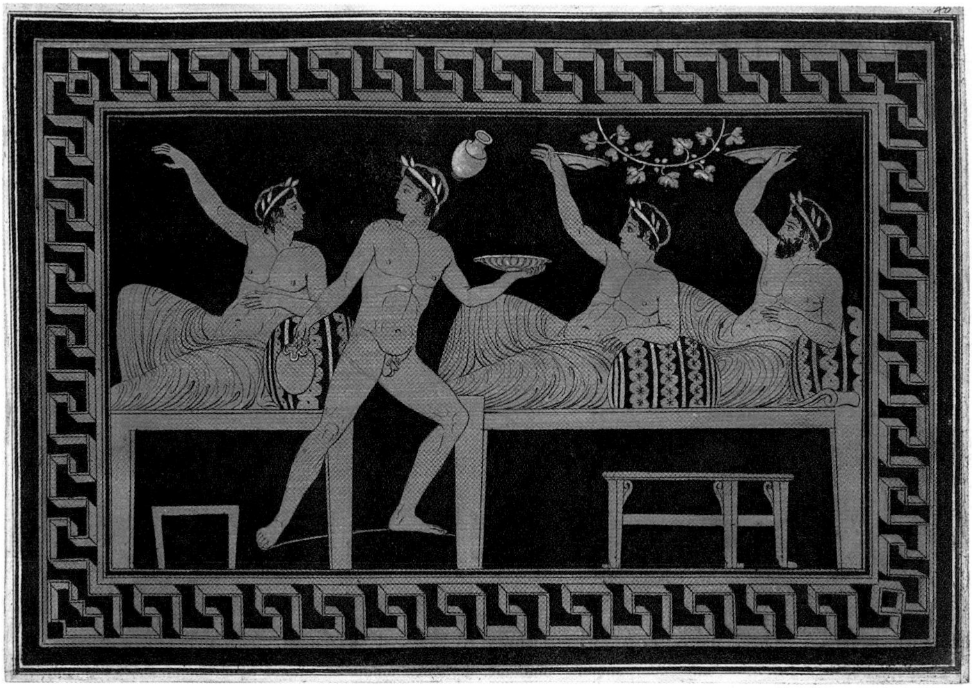

31. Greek men symposiuming it like it's 404 BCE. (Four men at a symposium. An eighteenth-century copy of an original Greek vase design. Wellcome Collection)

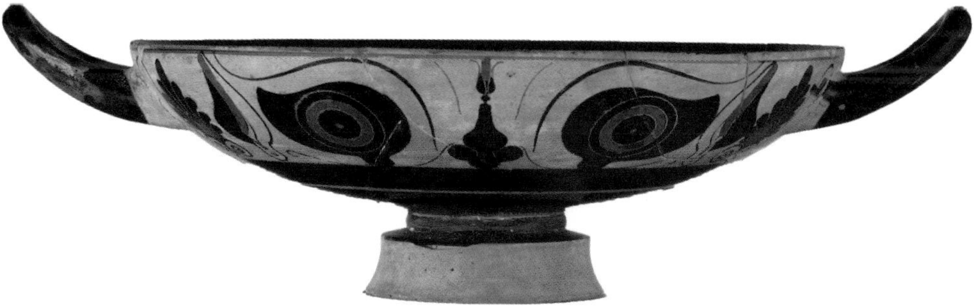

32. The kylix was a drinking cup especially designed to be difficult to drink from. (Terracotta kylix [drinking cup], attributed to the Group of the Phineus Painter Metropolitan Museum of Art, New York, USA)

33. A hetaerae plays a drinking game at a symposium. (A prostitute at a *symposium* taking part in some sort of drinking game, Attic Red Figure Kylix, attributed to Onesimos. Getty Open Access)

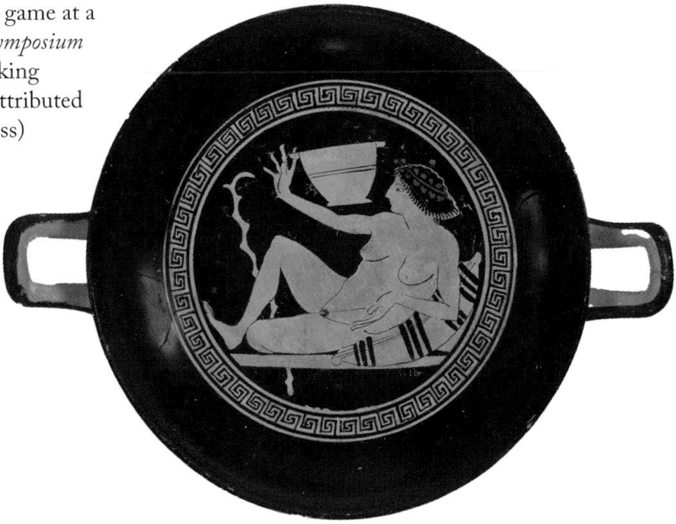

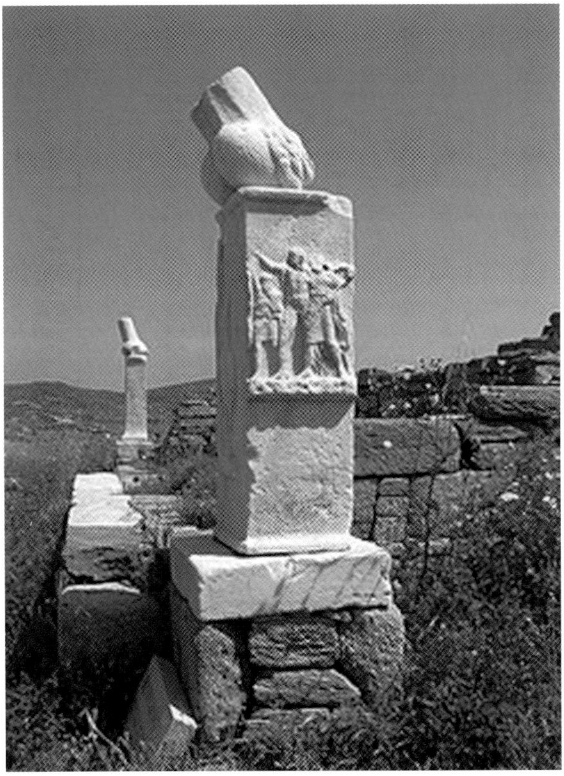

34. Two big knobs from Delos. (Phallus pillars in front of the Sanctuary of Dionysos, Delos shot by Anna Apostolidou. Wikimedia Commons)

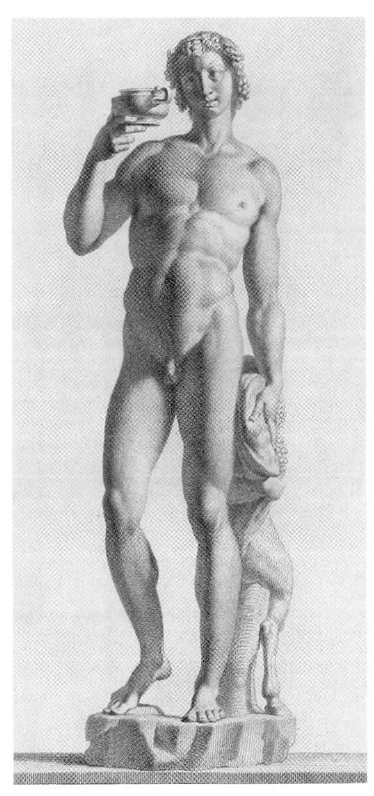

35. Dionysius, the god of getting pleasantly tipsy and ripping the limbs off youths. (Bacchus, from 'Museum Florentinum' [Statuae antiquae dorum et virorum illustrium]. Bequest of Mrs. Charles Wrightsman 2019, Metropolitan Museum of Art, New York, USA)

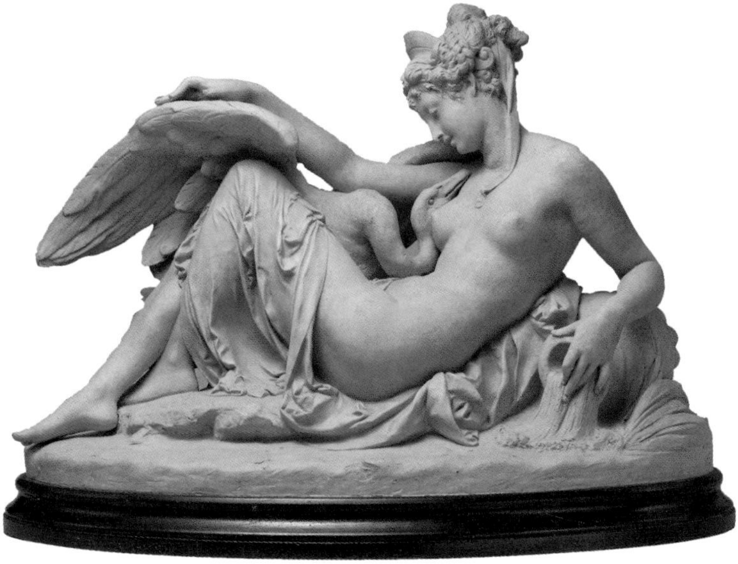

36. Leda and Zeus in swan form is a very popular image in antiquity, less so today due to the bestiality element. (Leda and the Swan, Albert-Ernest Carrier-Belleuse (French, Anizy-le-Château 1824–1887 Sèvres), Rogers Fund and Mr. and Mrs. Claus von Bülow Gift 1980. Metropolitan Museum of Art, New York, USA)

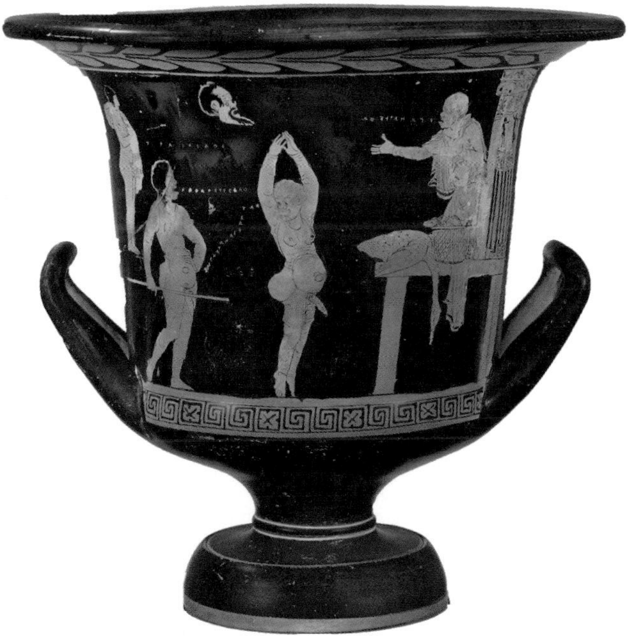

37. Vase depicting actors in costume; note the fake phallus hanging down. (Comic actors. Terracotta calyx-krater [mixing bowl] attributed to the Dolon Painter, Fletcher Fund 1924, Metropolitan Museum of Art, New York, USA)

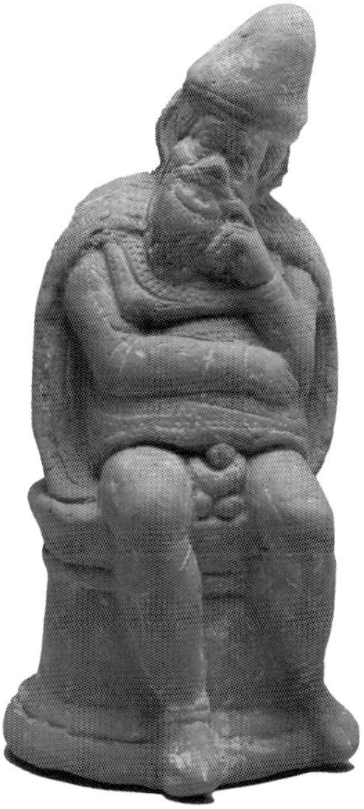

38. Terracotta statue of an actor, again note what's between his thighs. (Terracotta statuette of an actor, Rogers Fund 1913, Metropolitan Museum of Art, New York, USA)

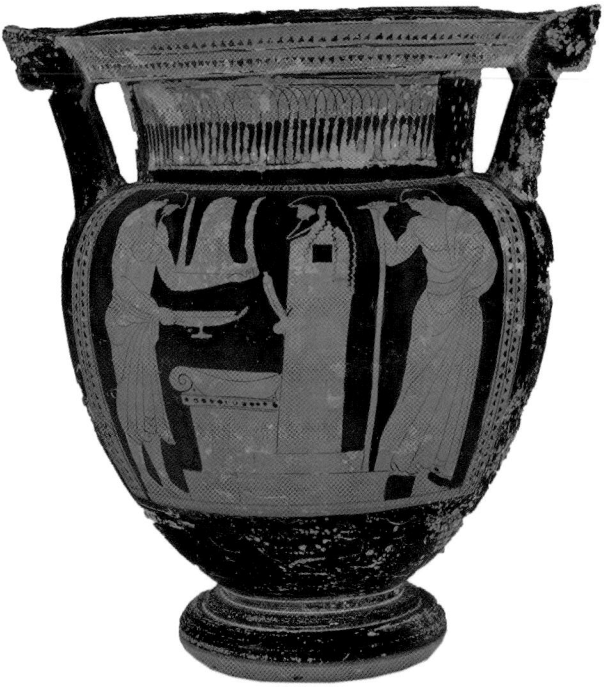

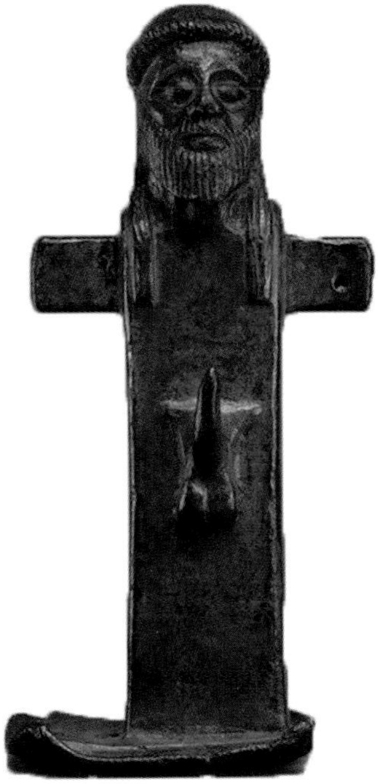

39. A Herm depicted on a krater vessel in which wine was mixed. (Image of a Herm. Attic Red-Figure Column Krater, Gift of Vasek Polak, Metropolitan Museum of Art, New York, USA.)

40. Bronze Herm. (Bronze Herm, Gift of Norbert Schimmel Trust 1989, Metropolitan Museum of Art, New York, USA.)

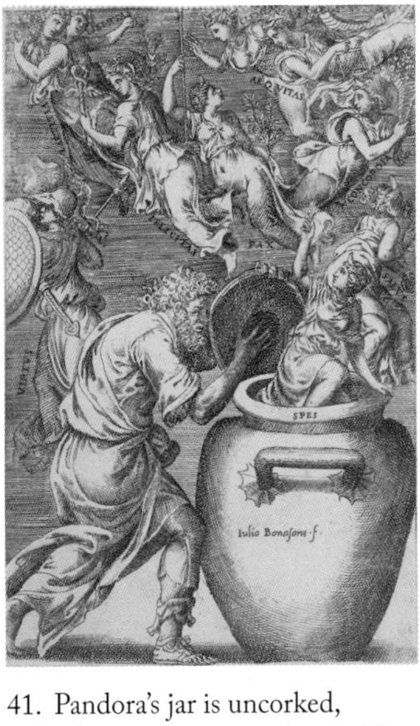

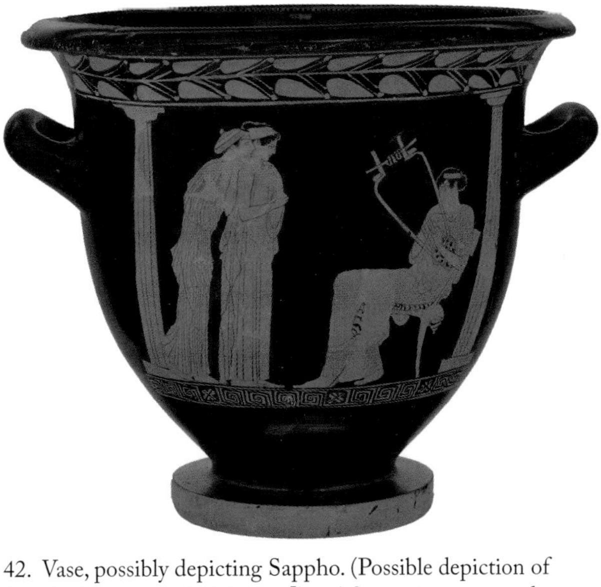

41. Pandora's jar is uncorked, unleashing calamity on the world. (Epimetheus opening Pandora's box, Giulio Bonasone, Gift of Harry G. Friedman, 1964, Metropolitan Museum of Art, New York, USA)

42. Vase, possibly depicting Sappho. (Possible depiction of Sappho. Terracotta bell-krater [bowl for mixing wine and water], attributed to the Danaë Painter, Rogers Fund, 1923, Metropolitan Museum of Art, New York, USA)

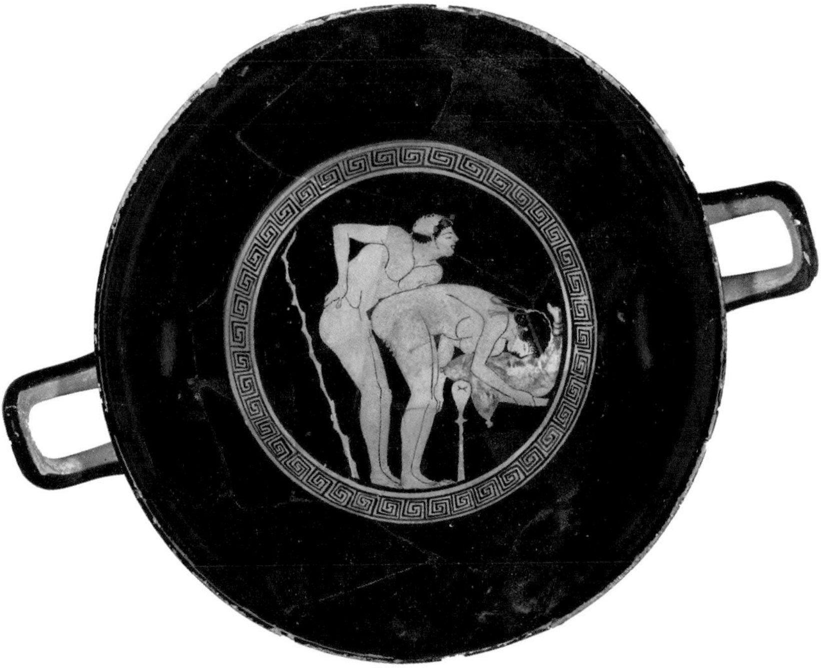

43. One of the milder examples of sexual imagery to be found on Greek pottery. (An erotic scene. Attic Red-Figure Cup, aattributed to the Foundry Painter [Greek (Attic), active 500–470 BC]. Getty Open Access)

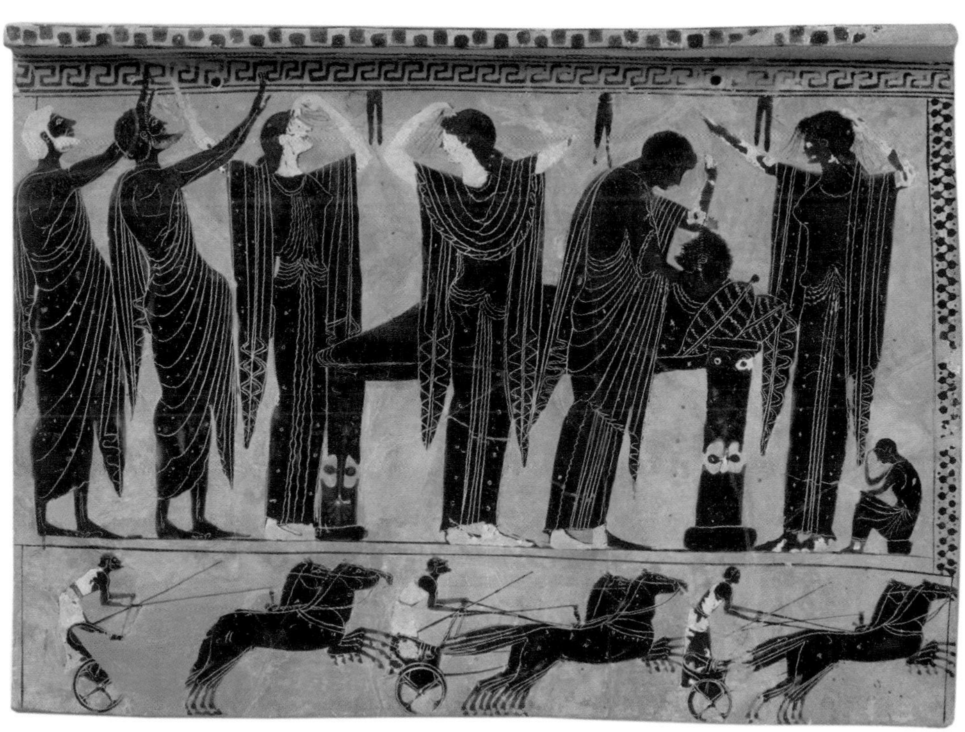

44. A funeral attended by both men and women. And apparently a stellar place to start an affair. (Terracotta funerary plaque, Rogers Fund 1954, Metropolitan Museum of Art, New York, USA)

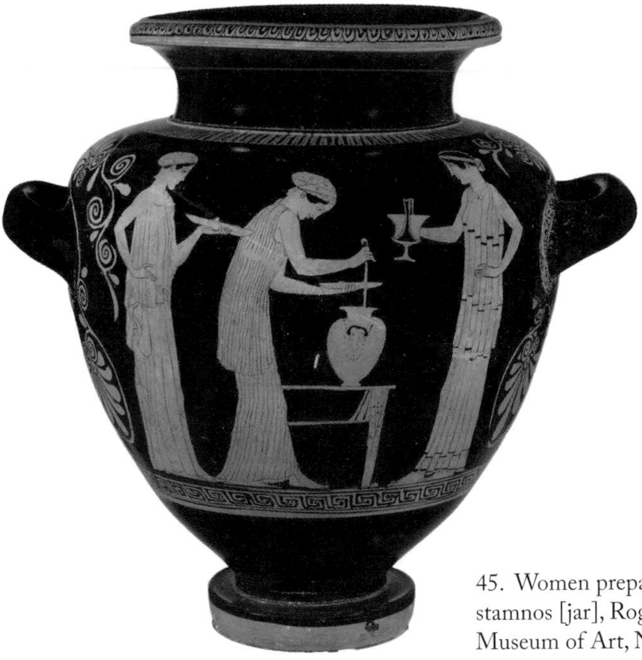

45. Women preparing for a festival. (Terracotta stamnos [jar], Rogers Fund, 1921 Metropolitan Museum of Art, New York, USA)

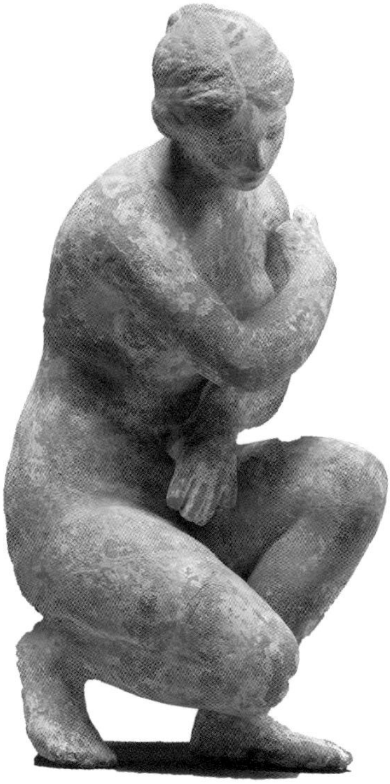

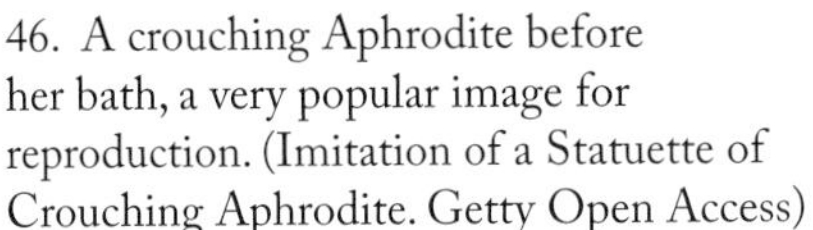

46. A crouching Aphrodite before her bath, a very popular image for reproduction. (Imitation of a Statuette of Crouching Aphrodite. Getty Open Access)

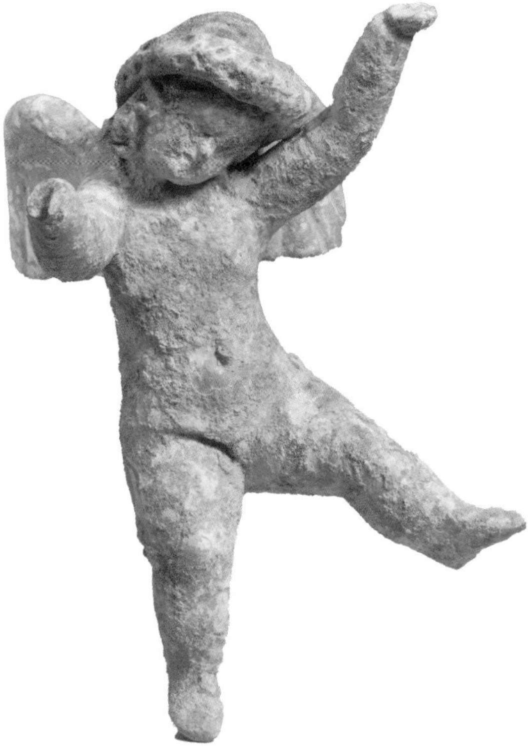

47. A deceptively jolly and harmless-looking Eros, hiding his dark nature. (Terracotta statuette of Eros flying, Rogers Fund 1911, Metropolitan Museum of Art, New York, USA)

beyond the dreams of every writer burning from the injustice of an Amazon one-star review.

Women reading this book are no doubt now all grinding their teeth and feeling really not very warm towards Hesiod, Semonides and Archilochus. We do, however, need to place our trio of women-averse poets in the context of their own times and perhaps that will illuminate quite why they are all so bitterly misogynistic. Perhaps. I'm not guaranteeing it will.

Chapter 10

Wives – Sharing the Burden or the Cause of It?

Hesiod's poem *Works and Days* is a guide to agriculture written in the seventh century BCE and it is very thorough in its advice: from when the best time is to plough the fields to the ideal age for a working ox (for those that must know, it's 9 years old), and onwards to what you should wear for winter farm work: 'lace on your feet close-fitting boots of the hide of a slaughtered ox … On your head above wear a shaped cap of felt to keep your ears from getting wet.'[1]

Hesiod also provides top advice on other subjects, such as how not to be a dinner party snob: 'Do not be boorish at a common feast where there are many guests, the pleasure is greatest and the expense the least.'[2] The correct way to urinate: 'Do not stand upright facing the sun when you make water … A scrupulous man who has a wise heart sits down or goes to the wall of an enclosed court.'[3] And which days are lucky for castrating cattle.

Hesiod, as you can tell from the above, is unsparing in the detail of what it was for men of his time to work on the land. He sees this as the noble profession of good men: 'Work is no disgrace, it is idleness that is a disgrace.'[4] Reading through Hesiod's lists of the best times to undertake the multitude of farm tasks that need doing, there's no getting away from the fact that it's a backbreakingly hard and exhausting job. Farming in the days before the invention of the motor engine was always hard but we know that it was specifically hard during the years that Hesiod was alive, the Archaic period.

Archaeological evidence suggests that populations were denser in urban areas during the Archaic era and there was an increase in the number of Greeks leaving Greece to found colonies on what is now western Turkey, both of which would suggest that populations were moving away from farming or away from Greece altogether. Making a living off the land had clearly become a much harder task, hard enough for significant numbers to give up on it altogether.

For those that did not give up, sell up and head for the cities, or a new hopefully more bountiful life overseas, assistance was needed for them to cling onto their way of living and their land. They needed a helpmate; they needed a wife. You'll be unsurprised that the Wikipedia of Archaic Greek farming, Hesiod, has plenty of advice on scoring a wife too.

Hesiod advises that men should marry when they are 'not far short of thirty years'.[5] This is such good advice that Plato, writing three hundred years later than Hesiod, still holds by it, stating that 30 to 35 is the ideal age for men to marry. Who knows, perhaps Plato also adhered to Hesiod's advice on cattle castrating and how to pee correctly too, good advice is good advice.

Hesiod continues:

> Marry a maiden so you can teach her careful ways and especially marry one who lives near you but look well about you and see that your marriage will not be a joke to your neighbours. For a man wins nothing better than a good wife and again nothing worse than a bad one, a greedy soul who roasts her man without fire strong though he may be and brings him to a raw old age.[6]

Much as firsthand experience informs his detailed tips on running a farm, the same was likely true of his advice on women and marriage, which make for interesting speculation on Hesiod's private life.

The wife's role in managing her husband's outgoings is the anxiety that is lurking behind much of Hesiod's advice. It's also lurking behind those nasty words of Semonides. 'Of work the only thing she knows is eating, And when the god sends an evil winter she is too lazy to pull her chair near to the fire.'[7] This reads differently once we place it in its seventh-century BCE context, choosing the wrong animal type of woman could destroy everything a man had worked so hard for in such harsh conditions.

However, this antipathy and suspicion against women isn't just a feature of hard times in Greece, it is present even in the best of times such as fifth-century BCE Athens.

Athenian wives

> Of course you don't suppose that lust provokes men to beget children when the streets and the stews are full means to satisfy that? We obviously select for wives the women who will bear us the best children.[8]

Wives were for bearing children and for looking after the home. The importance of a wife is spelled out by the fifth-century BCE Greek writer and soldier, Xenophon, who puts them in the mouth of his friend, the philosopher Socrates:

> I think that a wife who is a good partner in the household contributes just as much as her husband to its good; because the incomings for the most part are the result of the husbands' exertions, but the outgoings are controlled by the wife's dispensation. If they both do their part well the estate is increased.[9]

We saw in Hesiod that wives held an important role in the fortune or ruin of the household; however, Xenophon, writing in the fifth century BCE, is a little more sympathetic than our Archaic poets towards women's role in the household. Quoting his friend Socrates (which he often does), he says, 'I can also show you that husbands differ widely in their treatment of their wives, and some succeed in winning their cooperation and thereby their estates, while others bring utter ruin on their houses by their behaviour to them.'[10]

Whereas Hesiod and the unpleasant Semonides blame bad apple women for a downturn in their husband's fortunes, Xenophon/Socrates see the blame as falling on the husbands.

> 'When a sheep is ailing,' said Socrates, 'we generally blame the shepherd and when a horse is vicious, we generally find fault with the rider. In the case of a wife, if she receives instruction in the right way from her husband yet does badly, perhaps she should bear the blame but if the husband does not instruct the wife in the right way of doing things and so finds her ignorant should he not bear the blame himself?'[11]

Socrates is positively brimming with marital advice, much as he is brimming with advice on pretty much any subject you can think of. However, not everyone is a passive listener or recorder (in the case of Plato and Xenophon) of our philosopher's wisdom. This being Athens at the height of his democracy, every man had a voice and every word he spoke was open to be challenged, even those of Socrates. Particularly those of Socrates because he doesn't half dish it out; the question is, can he take it?

> 'If that is your view, Socrates,' asked Antisthenes, 'how does it come that you don't practise what you preach by yourself educating Xanthippe, but live with a wife who is the hardest to get along with of all the women that are yes, or all that ever were or ever will be I suspect?'[12]

Ouch, dissing a man's wife is a blow below the belt, surely? However, Socrates handles it manfully by not immediately biting back, 'Well, your wife's face looks like the rear end of a horse,' to Antisthenes and instead says:

> I observe that men who wish to become expert horsemen do not get the most docile horses but rather those that are high-mettled, believing that if they can manage this kind, they will easily handle the other. My course is similar. Mankind at large is what I wish to deal and associate with, and so I have got her, well assured that I can endure her, I shall have no difficulty in my relations with all the rest of mankind.[13]

Proving that Antisthenes didn't need to insult Socrates' wife, he is quite capable of doing that job for himself.

Socrates is a man ahead of his time in believing that husbands should treat their wives kindly and that offering up marriage advice to your mates is a good idea and not at all likely to annoy them intensely. Writing hundreds of years later in a Greece that is now a colony of Rome, Plutarch writes an entire essay of advice to newlyweds Pollianus and Eurydice.

Plutarch's marriage advice centres on marriage being a partnership far beyond what we've heard from our earlier Greeks, their ideas around marriage are centred around the duties of the man and woman to maintain the *oikos*. Plutarch dishes out his advice based on what is still a key Greek pastime five hundred years after Socrates: philosophy. 'Philosophy weaves a spell over those who are entering together into a lifelong partnership and renders them gentle and amiable to each other.'[14] A sentiment which, although touching, wasn't the case with the most famous philosopher ever, Socrates, and his wife. One cannot imagine them ever being 'gentle and amiable' to each other.

Plutarch's marriage advice is all very sensible stuff, the stuff you can imagine any marriage counsellor dishing out in our day. He suggests trying to avoid disagreements and clashes in the early days of a marriage, which he gives a nice and very apt analogy for: 'household vessels as are made of sections joined together at the outset easily pulled apart by any fortuitous cause but after a time when their joints become set, they can hardly be separated by fire and steel.'[15]

He notes that the early days of marriage, when you can't keep your hands off each other and spend the whole time shagging, are not 'enduring or constant unless being centred around character'.[16] So basically, fall in love with the person, not their appearance or your lust towards them, which is such sage and sensible advice it deserves its own range of merchandise, including tea towels and fridge magnets. Elsewhere Plutarch advises men that marry above themselves to aspire to become better men, rather than 'try to humble their wives with the idea that they will have more authority over their wives',[17] that showing physical affection towards one's wife in public is not as shameful as airing 'recriminations and discriminations before others'[18] and comments that husbands 'who are not cheerful in the company of their wives nor join them in sportiveness and laughter, are thus teaching them to seek their own pleasures apart from their husbands'.[19]

Evidently there are some universal truths about making a marriage work that are as applicable now as they were 2,000 years ago, but there is also plenty in Plutarch's advice to the newlyweds that is unlikely to find its way into any twenty-first-century marriage guidance book. There's this warning to wives who use love potions and magic spells on their husbands that it is unlikely to bring them happiness but rather a 'dull witted degenerate fool'.[20] Or the suggestion that a wife should not be cross about her husband's licentious dalliances with a servant or paramour because 'it is respect for her that which leads him to share his debauchery, licentiousness and wantonness with another woman'.[21] Then there is this comment: 'The women of Egypt by inherited custom were not allowed to wear shoes so that they should stay home all day and most women if you take from them gold-embroidered shoes, bracelets, anklets, purple and pearls, stay indoors.'[22] I do know women who won't leave the house without a fully made-up face and their hair straightened, so Plutarch is not entirely wrong. Although as noted by Plutarch in another work of his, not having shoes didn't affect Spartan boys' ability to go out and about and fight wars.

All of which is a reminder, if a reminder is required, that the nature of men and women has not fundamentally changed from the times of antiquity except in the places where it very much has. They are like us, whilst not being like us.

One of the recurring themes on marriage is that it is a partnership, one in which the wife was as important as the husband, something which for Hesiod was frightening and which for Socrates had a practical solution; women needed training up to be wives. There is a reason why Socrates believed women need training up that's slightly better than women are awfully bad people going right back to Pandora, the one who started it all off. 'And you married her when she was a mere child and had seen or heard almost nothing. Certainly. Then it would be far more surprising if she understood what she should say or do than if she makes mistakes.'[23]

Greek wives were considerably younger than their husbands, Plato's ideal age for a wife is 16–20 years, with her marrying ideally a man aged between 30 and 35 years. Aristotle favours women marrying at 18 to men of 37 and lays out some of the reasons why he believes this, which are deeply depressing to the middle-aged. 'They are in their prime of life and the decline in the powers of both will coincide.'[24] Yes, he is really saying that women start to decline at age 18 and men at 37. His other stated reason for the specified age bracket is a lot more rooted in fact: women who have children too young, that is younger than 16, have a higher chance of dying during childbirth. He adds to this that women who marry young 'are apt to be wanton', which is surely a compliment to her husband for inspiring such wantonness in her. If men, in comparison, marry too young, 'the bodily frame is stunted'. Yes, the ancient Greeks believed sex was good for achieving a respectable height.

Another reason for the age gap, unspoken by Plato and Aristotle but they were thinking it very hard in their head, is that it was likely to give the man a chance to have established himself (moulding a youth or two into being model citizens along the way) and therefore able to support a wife and expected family. As we noted when looking at Hesiod, this was not an easy thing to do in a society where one bad harvest or lame animal could lead to monetary catastrophe. A new bride, however, did contribute to her upkeep in the shape of a dowry.

Dowries

Dowries were one of the things that the Athenian sixth-century lawmaker Solon (on whom more later) concerned himself with. 'In all other marriages he prohibited dowries; the bride was to bring with her three changes of raiment, household stuff of small value, and nothing else. For he did not wish that marriage should be a matter of profit or price, but that man and wife should dwell together for the delights of love and the getting of children.'[25]

Solon may not have wished that marriages were a matter of profit or price but that's exactly what they were. The higher the dowry, the more attractive and advantageous a marriage was, both for the new husband and for the bride's father. A daughter was not as useful as a son, she couldn't work and bring income into the household.[26] As the fourth-century BCE statesman and orator Demosthenes declares in a speech, 'for who would ever have taken to wife a portionless girl from a father who was a debtor to the treasury and without resources?'[27]

The higher the dowry, the more marriageable the woman. It is difficult to determine exact figures, but some scholars have made a go of it and calculated that the dowry offered in the event of a marriage ranged from 5–20 per cent of the father's entire estate.[28] In Athenian law, if a man died with no male heirs his fortune could be inherited by his daughters. A woman who had inherited her father's estate was known as an *epikleros*, or heiress, and they were highly desired in the marriage market.

Although allowed to inherit fortunes, the law stipulated that Athenian women couldn't sully their tiny little lady hands with the financial goings on of the estate they now owned. The *epikleros* needed to be found a husband who could dirty their hands with all this money. First in the queue for this position were the heiress's own male relatives, presumably because it was in their own best interests to preserve and build upon the family fortune. Even non-heiresses in Athens had their property matters taken care of by male relatives.

So important was a dowry that the Athenian state was known to bestow one upon the relatives of men who had served the state. This was the case with the daughters of Aristides. a hero of the Greek war against the Persians. 'And they tell how his daughters were married from the prytaneium at the public cost, the city bestowing the dowry for the marriage and voting outright three thousand drachmas to each daughter.'[29]

Even the girls of poor families, whose fathers were not war heroes, could be helped by the state. 'For as things are now, even if a girl be poor, the law provides for her an adequate dowry.' Although this kind benevolence is undone by the sentence that immediately follows with the caveat, 'If nature has endowed her with even moderate comeliness.'[30] Leaving us with the unpleasant mental of the daughters of the poor being lined up and judged in some kind of beauty contest. No doubt the men of Athens merely saw this as fiscal responsibility on behalf of the Athenian *polis*.

The handing over of a dowry might have provided some legal protection for the Athenian woman for it was proof that a marriage had taken place. We see this in account of a legal case, it's a not terribly glamourous dispute over the will of a man named Pyrrhus and a resulting charge of perjury against another man named Nicodemus. Nicodemus in the original will dispute case had borne witness that he had given his sister in marriage to Pyrrhus and that they had a daughter named Phile who therefore should be in line to inherit Pyrrhus' estate. The nephew of Pyrrhus disputes this, claiming that Phile is the child of Pyrrhus' mistress and thus illegitimate.

Amongst the arguments put forward by the prosecutor Isaeus, on behalf of the nephew, is the issue of a dowry. If Nicodemus' sister had been legitimately married to Pyrrhus after his death she would be entitled to her dowry back.

> I desire first to ask some questions. He has deposed that he married his sister to a man who possessed a fortune of three talents; what dowry does he allege that he gave with her?
>
> Next, did this wedded wife leave her husband during his lifetime or quit his house after his death? And from whom did the defendant recover his sister's dowry after the death of him to whom he has deposed that he gave her in marriage?[31]

Perhaps they were legitimately married, perhaps Phile is the rightful heir, but that absence of a dowry is something that casts suspicion on the tale and is brought up as a sharp needle to keep pricking Nicodemus' thigh with.

> Or, if he did not recover it, what action did he think fit to institute to obtain her maintenance or the restitution of her dowry against the man who was for twenty years the tenant of the estate? Or did he ever, during all that long period, go and make any claim upon the heir regarding his sister's dowry in the presence of any witness? I should be glad to learn what was the reason why none of these steps has been taken in favour of a woman, who, according to the defendant's evidence, was legally married.[32]

The not so much subtext as repeatedly spoken text is that no good, decent woman went into a marriage without a dowry.

With such large sums of money involved, you might imagine there were some unscrupulous bridegrooms who would happily dispose of their young, naïve bride's dowry on whatever they fancied; this being fifth-century Athens, probably gifts for that buff young man he'd spotted in the gym earlier that day. However, in Athens at least, there was some protection in the law to prevent this happening. An Athenian husband was compelled to support his wife from the income her dowry raised but the principal amount was not to be touched, meaning on her husband's death she would receive the full amount back again. With disease, illness and war rampant in this period and the likelihood of her being widowed high, this was important because it meant she could remarry. Remarriage was a necessity for an Athenian elite woman who had no other way of supporting herself. Similarly, if the couple were divorced the dowry would need to be returned in full to her family.

Another protection was the stipulation that the dowry had to be returned if the wife died childless, for it at least encouraged a full marriage rather than a sexless sham just to get hold of her money.

Although having gone through all the legal protections afforded an Athenian wife relating to her dowry, we should underline that she had absolutely no choice in who she married. Her husband was chosen for her by her father or other male relatives, and for the benefit of the *oikos*. What she felt about her potential husband was of no consequence to the proceedings.

This is worth thinking about when we remember the age at which Greek girls married, barely in their teens and to men who were often double their age.

A good wife

We have seen previously in this book that a good wife was one who managed the expenditure of the *oikos* and did so in a measured way to the benefit of the entire *oikos*. But there were other factors that went into a perfect wife.

'I do not hold the same opinion ala Thucydides. For he declares that the best woman is she about whom there is the least talk among persons outside regarding either censure or commendation feeling that the name of a good woman like her person ought to be shut up indoors and never go out.'[33] So says Plutarch, a Greek living under the Roman Empire quoting a fifth-century BCE Athenian, the historian Thucydides.

Plutarch is living in different times, Roman-ruled times where, although women are still very much inferior creatures with no role in public life, they are a lot more visible than the women of Thucydides' time. Roman women attended the theatre and the games, they accompanied their husbands to dinner parties, and they went to the baths. The Romans being distinctly less nude than the Greeks, Roman women could also attend athletic competitions. Historically too they are much more visible, you can no doubt reel off a list of Roman women such as Agrippina, Messalina and Livia. You'll find it much harder to come up with such a list for fifth-century Athens.

Partly this is because women are allotted no role in public life save for some religious roles which means they are absent from the public discourse that is everywhere in ancient Athens. When Aristotle says man is a political animal, he really means man, as in those creatures with testicles and penises as opposed to a blanket referral to mankind.

Aristophanes wrote a play entitled *The Assembly Women*, as we saw earlier, whose premise is that the women of Athens take over the workings of government. A savage critique on the Athenian government of the time, the central joke is that the politicians have made such a mess of it we may as well give women a go at running things. A comedic premises that was used and re-used well into the 1980s with *The Two Ronnies* and their spoof serial, *The Worm That Turned*. *The Worm That Turned* imagined a society where traditional roles based on sex were reversed. It was set in the then dangerously futuristic year 2012, when men had taken over the traditional wife role in the home and women were serving a jack-booted Doris Day in a fascist police state.

In both *The Two Ronnies* and *The Assembly Women*, the role reversal of the sexes is treated as intrinsically funny, something that likely is lost on anyone born after, say, 1990 when traditional gender roles become much blurrier. *The Assembly Women* also makes good use of props including more costume phalluses, what I can only assume are fake beards that are as gloriously bushy as Greek men are seen sporting on vases and some cracking lines like this one: 'We can make excellent speeches exactly because we are women! Better than any man can. They say that buggered youths make splendid orators, don't they? Now, do we women know about fucking or don't we? We're naturals, right?'[34] One has to wonder how that went down with an audience packed with men who had played the role of *eromenos*, did they wince in recognition or belly laugh? We sadly shall never know, although we do know that Aristophanes was wildly successful and not run out of town – so he got away with that gag.

What do Aristophanes' Assembly Women do with their power? They constitute for what reads like a communist state, with all wealth centrally deposited and shared out. But also they enact laws that force men to have sex with ugly women before they are allowed near the pretty ones, which takes up most of the gag count for the second half.

To be unseen, unheard is part, for Greek men at least, of what makes a decent woman. In the speech that we opened this section with, Plutarch is referencing the fifth-century BCE historian, Thucydides, Thucydides himself is referencing a speech made by the politician Pericles. The occasion at which Pericles delivers this speech is at the funeral of those Athenians who have been killed during the Peloponnesian War against Sparta. 'And, if I am to speak of womanly virtues to those of you who will henceforth be widows, let me sum them up in one short admonition: To a woman not to show more weakness than is natural to her sex is a great glory, and not to be talked about for good or for evil among men.'[35] There it is, to be not talked about, to be invisible as such was the mark of a good Athenian woman and wife.

A similar sentiment is found in a Sophocles play, *Ajax*, when the hero of the play declares: 'Women are only beautiful when they are silent!'[36] Similarly in the *Odyssey*, Telemachus tells his mother Penelope to get back to her loom, declaring 'speech will be the business of men, all men, and me most of all; for mine is the power in the household'.[37] Again, in Euripides' *Trojan Women* when Andromache has the recipe for the perfect wife, we find the same sentiment. 'I offered a quiet tongue and a gentle eye to my husband.'[38]

I'll leave the final word on the unspoken words of women to Plutarch, who manages to compare the female sex not only to small, shelled reptiles but also to musicians in the same analogy, which is masterful. 'Pheidias made the Aphrodite of Eleans with one foot on a tortoise, to typify for womankind keeping at home and keeping silent. For a woman ought to do her talking either to her husband or through her husband, like the flute-player she makes a more impressive sound through a tongue not her own.'[39]

Chapter 11
Women's Lives

'Er indoors – the seclusion

We have seen how for Athenian men an ideal Athenian woman was neither talked about nor seen, her role was in the home – quite literally. You will find lots in our literary sources on Athenian women being confined to their homes and rarely venturing outside. Such as this one: 'Nor do married women accompany their husbands dinners or think of dining with them in the company of strangers especially not unexpected guests.'[1]

Or perhaps this from Euripides: 'the husband when he's annoyed with the company of those inside can go and ease his heart's vexation. But we have to look to one person alone.'[2] The ideal Athenian woman, according to Aristotle, 'should allow none to enter without her husband's knowledge'. Not even her friends, 'dreading always the gossip of gadding women, which tend to poison the soul'.[3] A rule that is taken to absolute highest level in this deposition during a legal case: 'he came to my house at night, drunk, broke down the doors and entered the women's chambers where inside were my sister and nieces who have lived such modest lives that they feel shame at being seen by their own family members.'[4]

The idea that not only are women confided to the home but also a particular part of the home is something that pops up in Xenophon too. 'I showed her the women's quarters too, separated by a bolted door from the men's, so that nothing which ought not to be moved may be taken out, and that the servants may not breed without our leave.'[5] A quote that some have taken to mean that the women were locked into a single part of the house. Although the context seems quite clear, that the bolt is in place to stop the servants thieving valuables.

When women did go out, rarely according to our sources and never if they were extremely proper women, they wore veils, much in the manner of the modern-day burqa which obscured their features. As well as being silent, women were supposedly also invisible.

Controlling women – the law

Evidence of how Athenian women ought to behave is found outside of our male literary sources mouthing off, it features in laws too. Much of Athenian law had been gifted to it by a man who became known as Solon the Lawgiver. Born in 630 BCE, Solon's career took off when he was put in charge of the Athenian campaign against the Megarians. It's worth taking a moment to appreciate and indeed marvel at how he secured this job because it's really quite extraordinary.

Burning with shame at an Athenian measure designed to end the war with the Megarians, Solon wrote a poem that channelled this disgust and headed down to the marketplace.

> After a large crowd had collected there, he got upon the Herald's stone and recited the poem ... This poem is entitled Salamis and contains a hundred very graceful verses. When Solon had sung it, his friends began to praise him, and Peisistratus in particular urged and incited the citizens to obey his words. They therefore repealed the law and renewed the war, putting Solon in charge of it.[6]

Now that is the power of poetry! Or of an exasperated elite who, exhausted after those hundred graceful verses, sighed and said, 'OK, if you think you can do better, be our guest.'

Solon took up the offer and, according to Plutarch, Solon 'conquered the Megarians'. But also, according to Plutarch, precisely one line later, 'Notwithstanding all this, the Megarians persisted in their opposition and both sides inflicted and suffered many injuries in the war, so that finally they made the Lacedaemonians arbiters and judges of the strife.'[7] At which point the elite rulers of Athens no doubt felt terribly smug, although the smugness may well have faded since Solon's non-conquering 'made Solon powerful and famous'.[8] Although the gods know why. Trying to fight an enemy and not succeeding in crushing them to the extent that an independent panel have to decide who wins is hardly the destruction of Troy or Alexander the

Great's conquering. Still, this along with some other stuff that Solon did make him the go-to guy to sort out the difficulties afflicting Athens at that time.

The big-time difficulties that Athens was facing in this era included a whopper of a question: how should their city be run? 'The Hill men favoured an extreme democracy, the plain men an extreme oligarchy, the shore men formed a third party, which preferred an intermediate and mixed form of government.'[9] On top of this there were also bubbling away a lot of the issues that had made Hesiod so cross a hundred years before; the poor were at the mercy of the rich, with indebtedness common. In desperation and because they had nothing more to spare, the poor of Athens were putting themselves up as the collateral for their debts. The rich weren't hesitating from calling in that debt with the result that Athenian citizens were finding themselves enslaved, sometimes even sold to foreigners and shipped abroad. There is mention of people selling their own children to escape the financial mess they had found themselves in.

This is hardcore stuff, combustible stuff; a society brimming with desperate men at a point when discussions are underway as to how the state should be run. It could so easily have exploded into civil unrest and all the horrors that brings. That it doesn't is in a large part down to Solon, both his laws, and the type of man he was. Solon was the type of man who, when it was suggested to him that he install a tyranny as surely the easiest way to make all the reforms that needed to be enacted, replied, 'That tyranny was a lovely place but there was no way down from it,'[10] and then he went and wrote a poem about it. Of course he did.

Given the huge situation he was tasked with resolving, it's amazing that Solon found the time to make laws on how many garments Athenian women should wear.

> He also subjected the public appearances of the women, their mourning and their festivals, to a law which did away with disorder and licence. When they went out, they were not to wear more than three garments, they were not to carry more than an obol's worth of food or drink, nor a pannier more than a cubit high, and they were not to travel about by night unless they rode in a wagon with a lamp to light their way.[11]

People were selling their children, and this is what Solon concerns himself with? I am not alone in questioning Solon's laws on women, even his admiring biographer Plutarch here says, 'But in general, Solon's laws concerning women seem very absurd.'[12] Disclaimer inserted here, Plutarch is writing in a Greece that is five hundred years from Solon's time and now part of the Roman Empire. Which probably explains a lot of his incomprehension at Solon's measures towards women, Romans are very good on laws and slightly less oppressive over women. Although the Romans too found time in the second century BCE to bother themselves with women's clothing, the Lex Oppia forbade them from wearing overly colourful clothing and no more than an ounce of gold about their person. The Lex Oppia was not law for long – the Roman matrons, much in the manner one of Aristophanes' gangs of women in *The Assembly Women* or *Lysistrata*, worked together to get the law repealed and their bling returned.

Philosopher Plato was of the view that Solon's laws were not nearly controlling enough and came up with all manner of helpful suggestions of his own. These included fining men over 35 who'd neglected to get married and sucking away all the simple pleasures of Athenian life. 'Furthermore, the unmarried man will receive no honour or obedience from the young and he shall not retain the right of punishing others.'[13] I mean, what is there left in life without street urchins bowing before you as you pass and beating the crap out of them if they don't?

Plato's killjoy attitude extends to how he thinks weddings should be. 'Let the wedding party be moderate. Five male and five female friends and a like number of kinsmen will be enough. Extravagance is to be regarded as vulgarity and ignorance of nuptial proprieties.'[14] Plato has clearly been subject to the end result of one too many bridezillas recently because his other suggestion is that both groom and bride stay sober throughout – as if.

But Plato's desire to interfere in the private lives of the newlyweds does not end at forcing them to endure their joint families getting together without the liquid lubrication that makes such a meeting bearable, no, he has another zinger of an idea. 'Let there be a committee of matrons who shall meet every day at the temple of Eilithyia at a time fixed by the magistrates and inform against any man or woman who does not observe the laws of married life.'[15]

There is a certain type of woman, of a certain age, who you may accidentally stumble across should you inadvertently drop a sweet wrapper in the street or be responsible for packing up their shopping in the supermarket. They are possessed of opinions, opinions which they determine you should know, and they are more than happy to share them to your face whilst holding a smug, condescending smile that gets smugger the more useless you are in their eyes. You'll become very familiar with them when you have a baby. Plato's 'genius' suggestion is to weaponise these women. 'The matrons shall have also the power to enter the houses of the young people if necessary and advise and threaten them.'[16] Chilling doesn't cover it. Terrifying is the word. Truly terrifying.

What are these laws of married life that mobilised gangs of middle-aged women have been told to enforce? Plato is very concerned that men are leaving the home to attend men-only common meals. Don't even think for a second that Plato has sympathy for the wives knocking about the house on their own, because you'll only be crushingly disappointed.

Plato neatly fits into this rule this cracker of an assessment on Greek women: 'But the women are left to themselves, they live in dark places and being weaker and therefore wickeder than men they are at the bottom of a great deal more than half the evil of states.'[17]

Plato's biggest concern is with the begetting of children, and this is where he sees his matron enforcers playing their part. They are to supervise (for supervise read interfere in the life of) the young couple for ten years, at the end of which if the couple have not begotten children, they may, with the consent of relatives and the matrons, part. There's a question here, in fact there's several around the importance of producing children in ancient Greece (we'll pick those up later) but the one that's bothering me is how Plato envisages this working, because he doesn't get into the nitty grittiness beyond saying the matrons can force their way into the homes of couples and threaten them. I'm not a man, but I imagine that a group of irate ladies of a certain age breaking into your house and insisting you have more sex with your wife or they'll be back is hardly conducive to any sort of atmosphere that would beget children of any description.

You will be unsurprised to learn that Plato's desire to control the behaviour of others, as he himself admits, 'In a well constituted state individuals cannot be allowed to live as they please,'[18] extends to how the begotten child should be educated and onwards.

For Aristotle there was a grave example of what happened if the state did not interfere in the lives of women. 'This is what actually happened at Sparta; the legislator wanted to make the whole state hardy and temperate, and he has carried out his intention in the case of men but he has neglected the women; who live in every sort of luxury and intemperance.'[19] We'll look into the lives of Spartan women in the following chapter but it's interesting to note here the difference in the treatment of the Athenian lawmaker Solon and Sparta's great lawmaker, Lycurgus. 'But when Lycurgus, as tradition says, wanted to bring the women under his laws, they resisted and he gave up the attempt.'[20] Spartan women are described by Aristotle as mischievous, disordered, and greedy. Sound familiar yet?

Both Plato and Solon continue, if in a slightly less extreme way, those views of Hesiod and Semonides before them: women are tricky creatures who need both watching and controlling. Of course, the easiest way to achieve both of these aims is to keep women where they could be both watched and controlled: in the home. As bombastic orator and politician, Demosthenes says of women: 'We keep *hetairae* [prostitutes] for pleasure, female slaves to take care of us, and wives to give us legitimate children and to take care of our household.'[21]

The reality

In ancient Athens, the man's sphere of influence was the outside, the public one that was jealously guarded from women by restricting what buildings they could enter (certainly not the nude space of the gymnasium), which public events they could attend (certainly not the nude space of the athletic games) and what public roles they could hold (none, but it's got nothing to do with nudity.) The women's sphere of influence was the home, which was intimate and private.

However, it doesn't necessarily follow that because Athenian women faced prohibition in certain public spaces they didn't venture at all. This may well be confusing you, given I've spent the proceeding paragraphs quoting sources from the era saying expressly that women were secluded in the home. It's time to flick back to the first chapter of this book and the disclaimer issued about who our literary sources are: they are all men. Disclaimer number two: context is everything.

Take the quote earlier in this section about the womenfolk surprised by that drunken boy breaking down their door, the context of this quote is a trial concerning an attempted murder by a man named Simon. The words used are from the victim, who of course is going to paint Simon in as bad a light as he can, whilst portraying himself as undeserving of this assault, a citizen of such virtue and decency his womenfolk blushed in the presence of their own male relatives. It's hyperbole, an exaggeration for a very particular reason.

We need to treat our other sources in a similar way by considering the immediate context in which they were written, e.g. is it a fiction or non-fiction, philosophy or tragedy? Let us take Plato; his thoughts on the age at which men should marry, that everyone should be married and that bands of hatchet-faced matrons should intimidate newlyweds into having children are all from a work which details his ideal society. It's not necessarily the society he is living in, it's the society he wished he was living in. Similarly, Pericles' speech talks of 'womanly virtues', which does not mean that women adhered to them, just that in Pericles' eyes the most virtuous of women did, which could be the majority or a tiny slice of the women he knew.

Do we believe that every woman of Hesiod's time was a barn-stealing hussy who was out to deceive and bankrupt every hard-working Greek farmer? Of course not, and so we shouldn't believe that every woman in fifth-century Athens was as silent and invisible as the uniformly male writers tells us they were. As the academic P. Walcott puts it, 'we have no way of being certain how far social reality corresponded to the social ideal of female seclusion.'[22]

It will no doubt surprise many of you who live in developed and progressive Western nations that 50 per cent of resident doctors in Iran are female,[23] and that women make up the largest proportion of graduates in STEM (science, technology, engineering, mathematics) subjects in Iran, a whopping 70 per cent.[24] In comparison in the UK only 34 per cent of those studying STEM subjects at degree level are women, although women make up a comparable percentage of doctors as Iran, 48 per cent.

These stats are interesting because they contradict everything we think we know about women living in Iran, that they are dreadfully repressed, treated as second-class citizens and face greater restrictions on their lives than Iranian men. Which is entirely correct, Iranian women do have distinctly less freedom than British women as can be demonstrated by lifting just two laws from Iran's penal code.

Article 638 of the Islamic Penal code states: 'Women, who appear in public places and roads without wearing an Islamic *hijab* [veil], shall be sentenced to ten days to two months' imprisonment or a fine of fifty thousand to five hundred Rials.'

Article 18 of the Passport Law of 1973: 'A passport shall be issued for the following persons according to this article … Married women, even if under 18 years old, with the written agreement of their husbands.'

I could go further and quote to you the penal codes on marriage, inheritance and who is awarded custody of children. Spoiler alert, women get the rawer deal even with recent loosening of restrictions on women's ability to initiate divorce. Although I am usually dead against using analogies and comparisons from antiquity to make a point about the present (the past is not so much a different country as an entirely alien planet whose cultural baggage we do not share and so can never truly see through their eyes), there is a thread here that can help us cut through the endless scholarly arguments about how secluded Athenian women truly were. Modern Iran proves it is possible to simultaneously have a penal system designed to repress women, have a clergy and religious police force who continually bang on about the inferiority of women and yet still have highly educated women working outside the home in key professions. It's contradictory, it makes no sense, yet it exists and perhaps helps us understand Athenian society a little better; it's complex.

Away from the literary ideals of ancient Greek men, archaeological evidence presents us with images of Athenian women engaged in a variety of tasks that don't involve being locked in the house all day. A quick search through the Corpus Vaosrum database brings up images of vases depicting women at the fountain house, at weddings, attending to cults, worshipping, washing together, talking together.

Archaeologists have struggled in vain to identify or even distinguish between sections of houses as being exclusively for men or women. Certainly, there was a man's area of the home, known as the *andron* where he hosted his *symposium* with activities that were probably best off kept sectioned a long way away from anybody else in the house.

Similarly, there probably were areas of the home where the women took precedence, where their looms were set up for weaving, for example. But they probably weren't as definitive as our sources would like us to believe. Because, remember, they are all men, the world which they project is likely one composed of the ways things were and the way they felt things should be. As well as a bit of saving face that their womenfolk weren't gadding about all over the city.

It is in an account of a murder trial, surprisingly, that we get a more nuanced account of how controlled the movements of Athenian women were and even an answer to the perplexing question of whether there really were women-only sections of the home.

The revelations in the murderer's defence

> Now Athenians, when I decided to get married and brought a wife into my house, for some time I did not wish to impose upon her or let her be too free to do whatever she wanted. I used to keep my eye on her as far as I could and give her a suitable amount of attention. But from the time my son was born I began to have more confidence in her and I gave her full responsibility for my house, as I believed this to be the best type of domestic arrangement.[25]

So begins Euphiletos, defending himself from the charge of having murdered his wife's lover, Eratosthenes.

Naturally he is going to paint himself in the best possible light, but the best possible light here is being kind to his new wife, trusting her with household affairs and slowly letting go of both his paranoia and restrictions on her. A good decent husband, a good decent man trusted his wife and did not watch over her movements the whole time. True, it turns out Euphiletos was dreadfully wrong in that trust because Mrs Euphiletos (who significantly isn't ever named in the text) abused his trust in the worst way possible, by having an affair.

So how does this affair start? Unless Euphiletos has a sexy doorman or visiting relative, our literary sources would have it that she would have no opportunities for such philandering because good, elite women never leave their domestic sphere. Except Mrs Euphiletos does and it is when she does that she meets the man she is going to be seduced by. It is at the most unlikely of venues that Mrs Euphiletos meets Eratosthenes, aka Mr Lover Man, I defy you to guess where, because it is the absolute last place and occasion you would ever think sexy feelings would bubble upwards: her mother's funeral. It is here Eratosthenes and Mrs Euphiletos spot each other, although no, they don't completely disrespect her mother by going at it then and there. We are told that Eratosthenes, 'by keeping watch for the times our slave girl went to market and by propositioning her: he corrupted her.'[26]

Although I can sort of believe that Eratosthenes is the sort of man who might well hang around funerals looking for vulnerable women to exploit, this meeting feels entirely unlikely, what kind of chat-up line is this to get a married woman to break her chastity with you? 'Hi, remember me, Eratosthenes? We met at that funeral, and I couldn't help but notice how damn gorgeous you looked as you sobbed and wailed at the death of the only mother you'll ever have. Fancy meeting up for a shag?'

More likely this is Euphiletos painting himself again as the perfect husband who had no doubts about his perfect new wife because she would only leave the homestead for something as important as her mother's funeral. It also paints Eratosthenes as having the blackest of hearts, for what kind of a man would seduce a woman at her mother's funeral! One fully deserving of being murdered.

For all we know, Mrs Euphiletos was knocking round the market most days and that is how the affair began, that certainly feels more likely than at a funeral but Euphiletos, as he says himself, is 'in danger of losing my life, my property and everything else'.[27] He needs the jury to be fully on his side. 'I would be very grateful gentlemen if you judged me as you would judge yourself were you to go through the same sort of experience.'[28]

The gentlemen of the jury were likely as shocked as you and I are at a romantic liaison being initiated at a funeral of a close relative, but matters were going to get even more shocking for those gentlemen because the affair itself was conducted in Euphiletos' own home! And not only when he was away on their farm but sometimes when he was present in the house!

Euphiletos talks here about men and women's quarters. 'I have a modest two-storey house, which has equal space for men and women's quarters on the upper and lower floors,'[29] but it becomes clear that these are loose terms. 'When our child was born its mother nursed it, and so that she would not risk a fall on her way downstairs whenever the baby needed bathing, I took to living on the upper level while the women lived downstairs. From that time, then, it became such a regular arrangement that my wife would often go downstairs to sleep with the child to nurse it and stop it crying.'[30]

Euphiletos' womenfolk, his wife and the slave girl, aren't confined downstairs to some specially designated zone, it's a convenience for Euphiletos because he gets a good night's sleep and doesn't have to deal with a crying baby and it's a convenience for Mrs Euphiletos not to have to keep getting out of bed every two hours in the cold and shuffle down a flight of stairs to stick an infant to her boob and then shuffle back upstairs again. It is all very practical and sensible, so practical and sensible that Euphiletos 'never had any cause for concern'.[31]

Might this be how we think of men's and women's spaces within an Athenian home, interchangeable according to domestic requirements, rather than rigidly policed areas? Perhaps Euphiletos had a room that served as his office on that upper floor he didn't particularly like his wife entering lest she muck up his filing, a space that might also be used to receive visitors in or for some other function. Euphiletos claims his house is modest, he had to utilise the space as best he could, although he never foresaw his downstairs area being used for passionate sex. He was under the impression that sex was strictly an upstairs pastime, perhaps with the slave girl, something his wife certainly suspects. 'When I got annoyed and ordered her to leave, she said, "Yes, so you can have a go at the young slave here. You made a grab at her before you were drunk."'[32] To our eyes this reads like Euphiletos' perfect husband mask is beginning to slip; however, given this is information Euphiletos freely offers in his defence, more likely drunken groping of slave girls is an inconsequential detail for the jury listening.

What is clear from Euphiletos' defence is that he wishes to portray himself as a hopeless sap of a man deceived by a serial adulterer. 'Eratosthenes from the deme of Oea who is responsible for this he has not only seduced your wife but many other women too. It's his specialty.'[33] The message to the jury is clear, it could've been your wife next. I've done the entire city a favour with my brutal murdering of an unarmed, pleading man.

I've said throughout this section that this is Euphiletos' defence against a charge of murder, but it's not what we think of as a murder defence. Euphiletos freely admits that he murdered Eratosthenes, he could hardly say otherwise when he'd personally gathered together a group of his neighbours to watch him commit the murder, even stopping off to take 'torches from the nearest inn'.[34] All the better to illuminate the murder for the chosen witnesses.

Euphiletos is defending his actions using an Athenian law that allowed a husband who caught his wife committing adultery with another man to kill his wife's lover or, less dramatically, demand a financial settlement off him. Euphiletos needs witnesses, not only to back up his assertion that Eratosthenes was banging his wife by catching them mid-banging but also that the financial settlement option had been raised. Eratosthenes apparently 'begged and pleaded not to be killed and was ready to pay the money at my recompense'. However, as Euphiletos bluntly puts it, 'I did not agree with his offer.'[35] He had the witnesses on hand to confirm that rejection and thus prove that Euphiletos had kept within the law.

Eratosthenes' surviving family clearly disagreed with Euphiletos' account of events, which is why Euphiletos is on trial, despite the efforts he took to make sure his murder was legal. Euphiletos' defence occasionally hints at how Eratosthenes' family viewed what had happened. 'He was not snatched from the street … as these people claim.'[36]

That the *polis* accepted the murder of one of its citizens for adultery, although with strong conditions attached, shows just how strongly they felt about extra-marital relations. That strength is shown by an extension of the law. 'Moreover, the lawgiver so strongly believed this to be the right course of action in the case of married women that he imposed the same penalty even in the case of mistresses, who are worth less than wives.'[37]

What happened to the woman caught in with her lover? The law stated that any woman caught in the act with a male lover could legally be sold by her male guardian into slavery. Although, unlike the killing or financial settlement required of the male party in this love fest, there aren't any examples of women being sold into slavery recorded.[38] Eratosthenes, the serial adulterer, is the criminal in this case; Mrs Euphiletos is the passive victim of his seduction.

Another however enters the story here, for although Mrs Euphiletos is not punished by being killed by her husband, as her lover is, as an adulterous woman, and with witnesses to prove this, the law compelled her husband to divorce her. A woman convicted of adultery was 'not allowed to participate in public ceremonies, nor wear jewellery and the most severe deprivation was probably that she would be a social outcast and never find another husband'.[39] It might seem a much lesser punishment than being murdered but women in ancient Athens were dependent on men providing for them; the divorced and disgraced faced a difficult future, one that might see them at risk of starvation out on the streets.

Euphiletos' defence is a rich document for revealing how Athenian husbands and wives truly lived together, rather than how Athenian men felt they should do so. Although we have to be just as careful with our source material given its context. However, revealed between the lines of Euphiletos' account of how he came to murder his wife's lover there is another story bubbling away that also offers up key evidence of how Athenian women lived. It's the story of the slave girl.

'Er not indoors – the lives of non-elite Athenian women

In Euphiletos' defence it's the slave girl who facilitates the affair that leads to Eratosthenes' death, it is she who he approaches at the market to get messages to Mrs Euphiletos, revealing a truth: not every class of Athenian woman was lumbered with an ideal that stated she should stay at home. Slave girls were sent out to do the shopping, draw water from the well and other such errands as she should be required to undertake, as did working-class women and women who had been freed from slavery. They also went out to work, holding down jobs, because they had to. Poorer households needed as many of their members as possible to bring in an income purely to survive and that included their women.

We know that Athenian women ran stalls in the market just as men did, because they are included in a law quoted by Demosthenes which made it a crime for 'anyone who makes business in the market a reproach against any male or female citizen shall be liable to the penalties for evil-speaking'.[40] Elsewhere in the same speech, the defendant's mother is said to have been 'a vendor of ribbons'.[41] This same mother has also worked as a nurse, 'you will find today many Athenian women who are serving as nurses I will mention them by name if you wish,'[4] the defending lawyer remarks.

Alongside nurses we also find Athenian women working as washerwomen, in the fields undertaking agricultural work, as wet nurses and midwives and as skilled musicians of the flute and harp. None of these are likely to have been from wealthy elite families, although there might be an occasion when this became necessary, as with the case of a man named Aristarchus.

Seeing Aristarchus looking a bit on the glum side, his friend Socrates commented, 'Aristarchus you seem to have a burden on your mind. You should let your friends share it, possibly we may do something to ease you.'[43] Which was the opening Aristarchus needed to have a bit of a bitch. A revolution in the nearby city of Piraeus had led to a flurry of Aristarchus' female relatives fleeing to his front door, 'sisters, nieces, cousins so that we are fourteen in the house not including slaves,' he complains, going on to note how little he makes from his land because the enemy have seized it, that his properties have no buyers and he can't get a loan from anyone. 'It's hard to let one's people die but it is impossible to keep so many in times like these,' says Aristarchus, who seems to have a hit list prepared in his head of which of his cousins, sisters or nieces are going to get it first.

Socrates listens to Aristarchus' intention to let his near relations die with surprising restraint before offering up the obvious solution.

> 'What about men's and women's cloaks, skirts, capes, socks?'
> 'Yes, all of these things too are useful.'
> 'Then don't the members of your household know how to make these?'
> 'I believe they can make all of them.'
> 'Don't you know then that by manufacturing one of these commodities, namely groats, Nausicydes keeps not only himself and his family, but large herds of swine and cattle too.'[44]

Having had capitalism explained to him, Aristarchus has an objection. 'But my household is made up of gentlefolk and relations!' The obvious retort to this is, 'Well, beggars can't be choosers,' but this is Socrates and the fifth century BCE so this point is laboured over many lines, lines which are pretty revealing in how different attitudes were back then. Today even your blue-blooded aristocrat will willingly open the doors to their home to the general public and set up a gift shop, garden centre and café in the grounds of their country estate if it'll allow them to hang onto said estate. The Duchess of Devonshire, a pioneer of this approach, manned the gift stall herself after her husband inherited a dukedom and a (then) crumbling Chatsworth House.

In comparison, Socrates spends quite some time convincing Aristarchus that commerce is a better course than letting your sisters starve to death. His arguments centre around the improvement of the household atmosphere, since by exerting his authority over them and making them work they will feel less of a burden and he will be happy with the money they bring in. 'To be sure to do something disgraceful, death would be a better fate. But the point of fact the work they understand is, as it appears, the work considered most suitable for a woman.'

Aristarchus takes onboard Socrates' advice and reports back that the women worked during dinner and only stopped at supper. 'They were happy instead of gloomy faces, suspicious looks were exchanged for pleasant smiles. They loved him as a guardian and he liked them because they were useful.'[45] By which we might conclude that thank the gods Aristarchus happened to bump into Socrates that day, otherwise a household tragedy may well have occurred. We may also conclude that elite women are so very dependent on their male relatives to support them, and that generally most ancient Greek men weren't like Socrates. The idea of elite women working with their hands for money was so deeply shameful for both the male guardian unable to provide for them and the womenfolk themselves that dying was a possible and expected alternative.

Like so much of ancient Greek culture, we are left with conflicting evidence on how constrained women's lives were in fifth-century BCE Athens. The legal system had several laws aimed at directly controlling the behaviour and movement with women, our male literary sources parrot the notion that women should be neither seen nor heard and it's clear that this was the case for some women. Yet we also possess evidence that flatly contradicts this. Socrates' wife Xanthippe, by all accounts of her, was no demure, silent, obedient wife. We have evidence of women holding down jobs, of conversing with men and that conversing being sought out by men, they also feature in visual arts doing things outside the home such as having a good gossip by the water fountain. It is fair to say women's position in Athens was complex and not easily placed in one box marked 'oppressed, stays at home but only in rooms dictated that she may by her almighty powerful husband', much as Athenian males may have wished this.

Later in Greek history, the women of Athens found themselves with more rights as their city was incorporated into the Roman Empire. In Roman laws, women could own property, dispense with a male guardian over seeing her financial affairs if she gave birth to three children, attend events at the amphitheatre (although women were segregated out to the crappier seats at the back along with slaves), theatre and races, and are generally much more visible in society. Although Roman women, like Greek women, have fewer rights than men.

Chapter 12
Women Outside of Athens

Unsurprisingly there is a lot less detail on how women were treated in the other Greek states, aside from Sparta, which we shall be looking at shortly. But what we do know is that although women were treated as second-class citizens, if allowed to be citizens at all, their status does vary from region to region and certainly between time periods.

Bull leapers and law keepers

We begin our tour of women's rights in the bits of Greece that aren't Athens with the Minoans. You'll remember the Minoans from the first chapter of this book, they were one of the earliest flourishings of ancient Greek culture whose civilisation burnt brightly from around 2000 BCE to 1100 BCE on the island of Crete. You will also possibly remember that what we think we know about Minoan civilisation comes largely from the British archaeologist, Sir Arthur Evans, whose findings from his excavations of sites, such as Knossos, were coloured by his own wishful thinking.

Amongst the evidence that Evans didn't get his hands on to inflict his own version of restoration, we do find a number of representations of women.

A Minoan rite of passage was bull leaping, which is exactly as it sounds, Minoan youths would line up and take turns leaping over bulls using a variety of acrobatic turns. From surviving frescoes, the execution of bull leaping looks not unlike the vault in modern gymnastics, if the vault had a head with very sharp horns, anger management issues and was charging towards you at great speed. I have a theory that we'd all discover our gymnastic potential in that moment, mine is fleeing for the nearest fence and throwing myself over it, landing in an ungainly heap in the mud. Not so for the Minoan youths, who presumably spent a lot of hours practising on the ancient equivalent of a vault before they were put in the path of the live version, you would hope.

What is interesting about Minoan bull leaping, aside from the fact that it ever existed as a sport/rite of passage (if there ever was an originator story it has been sadly lost to time, which I find unexpectedly irritating because I need to know if there were less popular, lower-league-type versions such as pig leaping or sheep leaping that weren't considered worthy of a fresco), is that it was undertaken by both boys and girls.

We find Minoan girls represented both as spectators to and participants in sporting activity, although the similarity in hairstyles can make it difficult to distinguish between the genders. The fresco which you will find referred to as the Akrotiri boxer depicts, depending on who you believe, two adolescent boys boxing, two adolescent girls boxing or an adolescent boy boxing with an adolescent girl. On other images from the era, we find women more distinguishable and distinguished with elaborate hair dos and wearing a lot of blingy jewellery. Minoan women appear as priestesses and hold positions in public administration. Arthur Evans uncovered enough evidence during his excavations to back up his belief that the Minoan religion was centred around the worship of a mother goddess figure; his mental leaps led him to tying her existence to Rhea, the mother of Zeus. Ignoring Evans' single-minded pursuit to prove the tales of Greek mythology as historical events, the artefacts he uncovered do indeed show what looks like the ritualised worship of a goddess.

We pick up the history of Crete a thousand years later with the city state of Gortyn and a very important inscription from the fourth century BCE. Why important? Because this inscription listed the law of Gortyn, including some interesting details on the status of women in the region. Rather handily the powers that be in Gortyn decided to inscribe these laws on the walls of their civic buildings where they were readily available to the (literate) members of the polis, and a number of these are extremely helpful to us in our quest to determine how women outside of Athens were treated.

In Gortyn, if a couple divorced, women were entitled to recoup any property they had brought into the marriage, but also half of any income that had been earnt from this property. Not only this, she also got to keep 'whatever she had woven',[1] which saved no doubt many a woman from staying longer in an awful marriage simply because she was damned if she was going to let him have that rug she'd been working on for weeks.

Should the wife die during the marriage, her property was similarly protected, with her husband being merely the trustee of what had been hers. Any action he wanted to take regarding his now deceased wife's property needed the consent of the children they had produced. If there were no children in the marriage, then the husband had to return to his deceased wife's extended family her property, half of any income derived from her property and also half of anything she had woven.

As in Athens, there is consideration given in law to heiresses, because the monetary stakes for both families are that much higher. Like in Athens, on the death of her husband, first dibs on her is given to the family. 'The heiress shall marry the brother of the father, the eldest of those living; and if there be more heiresses and brothers of the father, they shall marry the eldest in succession.'[2]

However, the legal minds of Gortyn are aware that forcing two people to wed by law does not always make for a successful marriage, and so there are get-out clauses for both the heiress threatened with marrying a family member solely so they can get their hands on her dosh, but also, surprisingly, for the sensitive male who might not want to marry her even though she is enormously wealthy.

> But if he do not wish to marry the relatives of the heiress shall charge him and the judge shall order him to marry her within two months; and if he do not marry, she shall marry the next eldest. If she do not wish to marry, the heiress shall have the house and whatever is in the house, but sharing the half of the remainder, she may marry another of her tribe, and the other half shall go to the eldest.[3]

If the husband should die during the marriage, she could keep her own property and 'whatever her husband may have given her',[4] although this was only permissible if these whatevers were written down and witnessed by three people who needed to be of age and free. There was to be no threatening your slave boys into falsifying documents to diddle your own children out of their inheritance. Or as the Gortyn code puts it, rather menacingly, 'But if she carry away anything belonging to her children she shall be answerable.'

These children mentioned did include daughters.

> The property should be divided fairly, and old the sons, however many there are shall receive two parts and the daughters one part each … And if should there be no property but a house the daughters receive their share as is written. And if a father while living wish to his married daughter, let him give what is written.[5]

What is most notable about the Gortyn code, aside from allotting property rights to women, is the emphasis on 'what is written'. You have to hope that there was a high literacy rate in Gortyn for husbands and wives to ensure they had scribbled down their every whim on who got what in the event of their sad demise. That the Gortyn code was inscribed and displayed on the columns of what was probably the main civic building in Gortyn shows how important they felt it was that citizens knew their rights. That it was inscribed on panels 30 feet high and 5 feet wide shows how important they felt it was that short-sighted citizens should not be excluded from knowing their rights too.

From all of which we can assume, I believe, a high level of literacy amongst the citizens of Gortyn and significantly fewer dodgy lawyers than perhaps elsewhere in Greece. By codifying and displaying the law in a public space, the power truly was in the hands of the people, including importantly women. No, they weren't in any way treated as equals to Greek men in Gortyn, but they significantly had access to where they stood in law and no disappointing husband could deny his soon-to-be ex-wife what was hers.

Women out of control – Sparta

Where Athens had Solon, Sparta had Lycurgus. Although, as we established in an earlier chapter, Lycurgus is a man much harder to pin down than Solon due to him possibly being entirely fictional. Nevertheless, for a man that might just be a convenient explanation for the oddness of the Spartan constitution, Lycurgus isn't half influential.

The laws attributed to Lycurgus touched on every aspect of a Spartan's life, including the production of little Spartans. 'He noticed too, that during the time succeeding marriage it was usual elsewhere for a husband to have unlimited intercourse with his wife.'[6] Which makes it sound like Lycurgus spent his pre-king years touring round Greece spying on newlyweds, because really, how else would he know?

The lesson Lycurgus took from his spying mission was not, 'aww how cute that those kids are so in love they can't keep their hands off each other', because 'the rule he adopted was the opposite of this; for he laid it down that the husband should be ashamed to be seen entering his wife's room or leaving it.' If you're thinking that's a hell of a strange route to take to encourage marriage and children, stay with me because there is a thought process behind this somewhat bizarre declaration. 'With this restriction on intercourse the desire of one for the other must be necessarily increased and their offspring bound to be more vigorous than if they were surfeited with one another.'[7] Right, if you say so, Lycurgus, although again I am wondering how he knows this, is he keeping a tally of when his pals have sex with their wives and then ranking their offspring as good Spartans or not so good Spartans? Lycurgus strikes me as a man who would have appreciated a spreadsheet and a good pair of binoculars.

Lycurgus had many other ideas on how good Spartans could be produced besides introducing the element of shame attached to men spending time with their wives. 'He believed motherhood to be the most important function of the freeborn woman. Therefore, in the first place he insisted on physical training for the female no less than for the male sex.'[8]

Elsewhere in Greece we find the likes of Plato and Aristotle offering up general guidelines on what they think is a good age range to get married, in Sparta there is no such thing as a general guideline for Mr Interference Lycurgus: 'he withdrew the right from men to take a wife whenever they chose, and insisted their marrying in the prime of their manhood, that this too promoted the begetting of fine children.'[9]

Lycurgus' obsession with 'fine children' leads us down some strange alleyways that seem at odds with the morality of the times. There was his proclamation that if contrary to his law, an elderly man should marry a young girl, it was entirely acceptable to move in a man in his prime into their home for the purposes of begetting those fine children. State-sanctioned threesomes, no less!

The begetting of those fine children by those prime men was made more attractive by Lycurgus' proclamation that if they didn't fancy it they need not get married and do the whole responsible family thing. They could 'choose a woman who was a mother of a fine family and of high birth and if he obtained her husband's consent to make her the mother of his children'.[10] We've had state-sponsored threesomes, now here is state-sponsored adultery! Imagine that in Athens, you can't.

It should be noted that despite the increased freedoms of Spartan women compared to women elsewhere in Greece, it is the men here who are being given the right to sleep with another man's wife. The wife in question is given no rights herself to introduce a better potential breeder into her marriage, nor, more crucially, the right to refuse one. The life of Spartan women at first glance appears far more appealing than the lives of Greek women elsewhere but there is a darkness lurking in the corners of what we are told, a darkness we shall aim our torches at, unflinchingly.

Spartan boys and men were the main target of Lycurgus's insane amount of law-giving, with every aspect of their lives rigidly controlled. The women in comparison get off lightly, sometimes in a bad way, with men given legal controls over aspects of their lives, but for once in the Greek world the spotlight isn't pointing directly at them and their behaviours and lives.

As a result, Spartan women are very different to the Athenian women we looked at in the previous chapters. They were not silent, mysterious creatures, they are given a voice and a load of pithy one-liners collated by Plutarch: 'Being asked by a woman from Attica, "Why is it that you Spartan women are the only women that lord it over your men," she said, "Because we are the only women that are mothers of men."'[11]

'One woman, observing her son coming towards her, inquired, "How fares our country?" And when he said, "All have perished," she took up a tile and, hurling it at him, killed him, saying, "And so they sent you to bear the bad news to us!"'[12]

There are many, many such examples like this and they are probably why Aristotle, at least, is of the opinion that Spartan women are a bit too much out of the spotlight and really that spotlight could do with being directly on full beam on them.

> In those states in which the condition of women is bad, half the city may be regarded as having no laws. And this is what happened at Sparta, the legislator

> wanted to make the whole state hardy and temperate and he carried out his intention in the case of men but neglected the women, who live in every sort of intemperance and luxury.[13]

Aristotle is firmly against women being allowed to make pithy one-liners, possibly because they are better than any he has ever thought up. He takes the relative freedoms of Spartan women to mean they are in control of their men, which obviously is a very bad thing in ancient Greece, the sort of thing that is so terrifying and unthinkable that there are comedic plays written on the subject so that the men may all work through those anxieties together in a safe public space.

We have looked at the education of Spartan boys in an earlier chapter and determined that at its kindest moments it could be considered child abuse and everything inflicted upon them would fall within what would be considered torture these days. Spartan boys were 'required to keep their hands under their cloaks, to walk in silence, not to look about them but to fix their eyes on the ground'.[14] Given the traumas they had suffered, including being kept half-starved, cold and subject to painful whippings, this feels like a natural response rather than another one of Lycurgus' damn regulations.

But their torment was not over with their boyhood, for when they reached that point of adolescence when natural feelings towards ladies start to emerge, Spartan youths were given 'a ceaseless round of work and contrived constant occupation'[15] to exhaust the teenage horniness out of them.

The lives of Spartan women with their exercising and competitive pithy one-liners is looking pretty damn attractive now, isn't it? Because Spartan men don't even have the luxury other Greek men had of getting pissed with their mates and letting off a bit of steam, because their version of the *symposium* is held out of doors, in public. 'The conversation at the public meals turns to great deeds wrought in the state, and so there is little room for insolence or drunken uproar, for unseemly conduct or indecent talk.'[16]

If you're thinking, yes, this may produce hardy, obedient soldiers but surely it's going to mess you up mentally big time, you're entirely correct. Spartan men, raised altogether, brutalised altogether and having had all their puberty hormones exhausted out of them via hard labour, struggled to adjust to suddenly finding themselves married to a member of the opposite sex they'd barely glimpsed up to now. The clues to this struggle are in the details of a Spartan wedding, which we covered earlier and which you'll remember involved the Spartan bride being dressed up as a man for her wedding night, with the added hint that the consummation of the marriage may also have been tailored for men used to having sex with men. 'It was the norm for maiden girls prior to their wedding to be dealt with as if they were boys.'[17]

Post-wedding anal sex, there was no cuddle or follow-up normal heterosexual intercourse. No, the bridegroom then returned to his usual quarters with his fellow men/soldiers and he would continue to do that for the entirety of his married life, visiting his wife furtively and with shame, as proscribed by Lycurgus. If you thought relations between Athenian men and women were messed up, Sparta not only takes the biscuit but the whole damn packet of Hobnobs and a cup of tea to dunk them in. The line that illustrates just how messed up relations between Spartan husbands and wives are is undoubtedly this one: 'And this they did not for a short time only, but long enough for some of them to become fathers before they had looked upon their own wives by daylight.'[18]

Chapter 13

What Little Girls Are Made Of

A great chunk of this book so far has been about how much Greek men saw Greek women as 'other' to them, others that needed to be controlled, silenced and confined because of their otherness. Nowhere was this idea of otherness more obvious than in a new field that the ancient Greeks would become synonymous with: medicine.

The unmistakable, and unmissable, physical differences between the two sexes has shaped civilisations for millennia and ancient Greece was no different. The additional strength of men made them the prime earner of the family (and carrier of heavy objects retrieved from high shelves) and this necessitated that they be absent from the home for periods of time. Further absences were required for all the wars that the stronger, more aggressive sex was conscripted into.

Women may be shorter, weaker strength-wise and less prone to go off on one against an enemy army, but they do have that neat trick of growing children in their wombs, pushing them out their vaginas and then producing food for them in their boobs. This tied them to the home, because in an era before effective contraception there was a permanent danger they might be shooting more babies out their vaginas at any moment and besides which there were already rooms full of babies who would make a dive for her boobs the second she opened the door. Those with a bit of money had the option of purchasing the services of a wet nurse who could handle the boob-feeding side of things whilst the wife was busy producing more heirs for the *oikos*.

Greek medicine was centred around the concept of the humours. There were four of these: blood, yellow bile, black bile and phlegm. Each humour has its own characteristic; blood was warm and moist, yellow bile was warm and dry, black bile was cold but dry, and phlegm was cold and moist. It was an imbalance in these humours that caused illness, or so the ancient Greeks believed.

Although the ancient Greek medical model of the humours was finally abandoned and replaced by the big brains of the Enlightenment in seventeenth-century Europe who developed a better understanding of how the human body functioned, you could argue it still exists today in the alternative/complementary medicine sector. Reiki is an alternative therapy where a practitioner holds their hands over their patient in order to aid the flow of their natural energies because '"stuck energy" can lead to pain and illness'.[1] You'll find similar claims made about acupuncture, apparently the causes of aggressive energy are that 'the organs are out of balance and our energy flow becomes stagnated'.[2] A lot of alternative therapies talk about 'rebalancing' the body, a concept that is at the heart of ancient Greek medicine.

In ancient Greek thinking, people got sick in the winter because conditions were cold and damp, which led to an excess of phlegm. An excess of anything tilted the delicate balance of the patient's humours, removing that excess phlegm would restore that balance and their health. An excess of phlegm as the cause of a cold, if I'm being honest, is far more believable than disease-causing creatures so tiny as to be invisible propelled at high speed from the nostrils of the infected onto their new host ready to multiply in greater, but still invisible, numbers. The world of viruses and microbes reads like the plot of a horror movie.

I perfectly accept the existence of viruses and microorganisms, because people that know about that stuff tell me they do, but if I were really determined to investigate for myself (which I'm not) I could easily get my hands on a microscope and sneeze on a slide. The ancient Greeks did not have the scientific equipment we take for granted, they could only diagnose what they could see and what they felt.

The climate affected the balance of your humours too, as did your age and sex. Children were considered warm and moist, young men warm and dry, mature men were cold and dry, and old men are cold and moist. Women, like old men, were also moist and cold and, according to second-century CE doctor Galen, 'for the most part stay at home'.[3] Which is a neat explanation for the restrictions on women's movements in ancient Greece – 'it's for the sake of their health!' Warm, dry young men had nothing to fear from being outside.

As well as being cold and moist, women possessed an additional characteristic that separated them from men and provided a neat explanation for the workings of the female body; they were porous.

The sponge

Biologically, according to the collection of doctors' notes known as the Hippocratic Corpus which were collated and copied into more legible handwriting around the fifth century BCE, women were cold and moist and porous. It makes perfect sense that women were moist, they produced fluids that men did not, such as menstrual blood, vaginal secretions and breast milk. This abundance of fluids could only be retained in a porous body. All of which makes the female of the species sound like a damp sponge left on the side of the bath that hasn't been properly wrung out.

It was the sponge-like quality of women that was responsible for menstruation. Menstruation is of great concern to Greek doctors; along with bowel movements, it is diligently recorded as having occurred or not occurred in patient observations. 'If menses do not flow women's bodies become prone to illness.'[4] Which you can sort of get if you think of women as being like a sponge, if you don't wring out a sponge not only does it become bloated and heavy, it will also eventually become mouldy. The Greeks believed that girls only began menstruating at puberty because before that point their passages/vessels were too narrow for the blood to escape from. They applied the same narrow vessel theory as to why boys only start to produce sperm at puberty.

Women's spongy nature was linked to her inactivity. Men were hard and firm because what moisture they had was lost during manual labour and poncing it out at the gym. Women kept at home, for their own good because the outside world was too chilly for their already cold bodily make-up, were just sitting around bubbling up fluids. This is also why women have breasts, according to Aristotle, 'and the area around the breasts rises distinctly in males also, but more so in females, for in their case on account of the abundance of secretions which descends the area around their breasts become empty and spongy.'[5] Women were one big water balloon waiting to pop.

Helpfully there was a natural process that dealt with women's heavy spongy state: once a month, their wombs filled up with blood which was drained away, along with other fluids that threatened a popping. This gave women at least one advantage over men: 'for the most part women do not suffer from haemorrhoids, nose bleeds or any other discharge unless the menses are suppressed,'[6] is one such bold claim. So bold a claim (statistically today with all that modern medicine has to offer, 40 per cent of pregnant women experience haemorrhoids) that the author immediately backtracks/hedges his bets with 'if any of these discharges do take place the menstrual flow is less in quality, as if the secretion is being re-routed to these'.[7]

The thing about Greek doctors is that you can occasionally get caught up in their logical fallacies – take this sensible pronouncement: 'the menses flow thickest and heaviest during the middle days while at their onset and finish they are lighter and finer.'[8] As a description of a period it's pretty spot on for the vast majority of women; clearly this Greek doctor has talked to many women about their periods and made careful notes of their responses. Although possibly not, as the very next line stated with similar confidence is: 'In every healthy woman the proper amount of menstrual blood flow is two Attic kotyks.'[9] Two Attic kotyks is equivalent to around a pint or 568 ml. If you've ever given blood, you'll know what a pint of blood looks like, it's a full bag. Women do not have full-bag periods, you'd need a mattress-thick sanitary towel to soak that lot up. The actual figure is between 25 and 90 ml of blood. The moral of the story is that even when Greek doctors are sounding at their most plausible, a fist full of salt is still required.

Once a girl began menstruating, it was essential that she kept doing so, unless pregnant, because if she didn't then the blood would build up in her body and cause terrible illnesses. What sort of illnesses? Those with a squeamish disposition, close your eyes now; pus expelling and tumour growing. There are a number of suggestions put forward on how to re-start a woman's menstrual cycle and keep it flowing, some of which I am fully on board with such as the theory that sexual intercourse heated the blood, which in turn would aid menstruation. Go forth, women, and shag for the good of your health! No, genuinely do. Gynaecologist Soranus notes that women who remarry after widowhood menstruate more freely and that virginity could be detrimental to the health of a young girl. Soranus is heavy on prescribing lots of sex for his patients. Other suggestions for bringing on menstruation sound distinctly less fun, such as purging. Purge is never a positive word.

A heavy menstrual flow was considered better than a light one because it was properly draining away those dangerous fluids that built up in women. Given that Greek doctors thought that a normal blow of menstrual blood was a full pint, I dread to think what they considered a heavy flow – a life-threatening haemorrhage, perhaps? Other symptoms that to us are extremely alarming, such as vomiting blood, are written off by ancient doctors as helpful for the woman in keeping her fluid levels down. The essential thing was that women got rid of their excess blood; any orifice, it would seem, would do.

The beast within

See if you can guess what Plato here is describing: 'when remaining unfruitful long beyond its proper time, [it] gets discontented and angry, and wandering in every direction in through the body closes up the passages of the breath and by obstruction of respiration, drives them to extremity causing all varieties of disease.'[10] It reads like some horrendous parasite the size of a snake, wriggling around inside the body.

What Plato is describing is a part of the female anatomy. One of the other things that distinguished women from men, aside from their sponginess and tendency to leak fluids from various parts of their bodies, was that they possessed a womb, a wandering womb.

Plato's wandering womb is an unhappy creature for it is 'desirous of procreating children'[11] and, unfulfilled, it causes chaos within a woman's body until 'the desire and love of the man and woman, bringing them together, and as if plucking from the fruit from the tree, sow in the womb, as if in a field'.[12] We are back to sex as a cure for disease again, which as previously stated I am all in favour of, as are Greek doctors. Apparently, the womb is moistened by intercourse, which is good because if it gets too dry it starts to contract and cause pain to the woman. Not only did this dryness cause pain, it had a terrible effect on the womb within them which would naturally seek out moist organs such as the liver, the heart, the diaphragm or the brain. You really did not want your womb suckering itself to them.

There were various ways to dislodge the womb from your organs such as the use of scents. Foul-smelling scents were used to repel the wandering womb away and sweet scents to entice it back into its proper place in the body. Which all sounds fairly innocuous, utterly inaccurate in its understanding of women's anatomy, yes, but at least having a bit of a sniff at some pleasant or unpleasant smells was unlikely to make the patient's condition any worse. Some of the foul odours used by Greek doctors, for example burnt hair, burnt wool, charred deer's horn, which were chosen because they all have the common denominator that they are hot, would have been administered via a treatment known as fumigation.

Nostrils weren't the only entrance routes to tackle that damn wandering womb of women, no, there was another one further down, a more direct entrance, let us say, a wider one, one that could stretch: the vagina. Fumigation involved a woman squatting or sitting on a stool over a heated pot so that the vapours could rise upwards into her vagina and cure her ailment or else add some additional ones to her original complaint. Fumigation, we are told, could take several days, which raises all kinds of questions for which I have absolutely no answers, not least to why one of the ingredients cited that was puffed up the vagina was a dead puppy.[13]

Dead puppy potions is the perfect point to introduce Soranus, a Greek doctor living in the second century CE who has the most sensible sentence in all of Greek medicine: 'the uterus does not issue forth like a wild animal from the lair delighted by fragrant odours and fleeing bad odours.'[14] It's about the only sensible advice he does give, aside from making sure you choose a midwife with nice short nails, which is supremely sensible given where their fingers are going to be headed repeatedly. Soranus is to be commended for demonstrating that, despite the basics of Greek medicine being our predominant understanding of illness and disease up to the seventeenth century, it was not an immovable set of facts. It was, as stated previously, a scientific method to which new theories and new ideas were added.

What we must bear in mind with all of this is that the reason Greek doctors were so clueless about female and indeed male anatomy was because they had never seen inside a body. There are mentions in our sources of Herophilius, a native of the city Alexandria in Egypt, born around 335 BCE, who dissected human bodies; unfortunately, his accounts of these dissections were lost when the Library of Alexandria famously burned down in 391 CE. I think it is fair to assume that the works of Herophilius were rarely taken out on loan since they appear to have had no impact on what the Greeks knew about our internal organs. It was centuries later that it became acceptable for doctors to study anatomy by dissecting human bodies. Our Greek doctors are making their assessments purely on what they can see externally, excretions and fluids. They have no access to X-rays or blood tests or MRI scanners or any of the other diagnostic apparatus we take for granted today. It's not surprising they got things wrong.

One thing they definitely got wrong was the idea that women were men but with their genitals inverted, men gone wrong, you might say. Galen describes how a man's penis, inverted, became the vagina of a woman, and his testicles mutated into ovaries. Again, you can sort of see where he is coming from, if you squint and use your imagination, but it is another cheap shot at underlining how man was the norm, women were the abnormal, their deformed version with crazy innards and leakages that men simply did not have.

Chapter 14

Men, Women and Sex

Wives, as we have seen, had two specific roles: the running of the household and producing heirs for their husbands. We have looked at the former of these roles and how much anxiety there was about choosing a wife who might not possess the skillset for running the household or, worse still, not be willing to learn how not to squander the hard work of her husband on fripperies. But a wife's other role of producing heirs created a fair amount of anxiety too for the Greek male.

There is a real fear lurking in the minds of Greek men that their son, the heir, might not be their son at all and the *oikos* had been infiltrated by another man's bloodline. This fear of being betrayed in the worst way imaginable by your wife is another reason why we find quite so many laws controlling the movement and behaviour of women. There is much mention of the importance of procreation in the works of the ever-keen-to-dish-out-advice philosophers of ancient Greece but what we don't find, however, is much in the way of details of how those legitimate heirs, or cuckoos in the nest, came to be procreated, marital sex in other words.

Our extremely thorough farmer poet Hesiod, who is happy to advise men on the correct way to have a wee, is strangely silent on the subject of sex. True, he does throw in the odd line here and there about the best days to 'beget' children. 'The ninth of mid month improves towards evening; but the first ninth of all is quite harmless to men. It is a good day on which to beget or be born both for a male or a female; it is never a wholly evil day.'[1] But he never goes beyond this into what sexual positions might be most useful for that begetting.

If you ever wondered how sex talk became known as 'the birds and the bees', might I put forward Plutarch as a possible originator for this piece of cracking advice for his honeymooning pals. 'Many of the newly married women because of their first experiences get annoyed with their husbands and find themselves in like predicament with those who patiently submit to bee stings but abandon the honeycomb.'[2] Which is surprisingly coy advice for a society that routinely depicted gang bangs on its crockery.

The rest of Plutarch's advice is similarly wrapped with the ribbon of metaphors and the bows of cute customs, such as nibbling a quince before hopping into bed together for a sweeter experience. Nowhere does he suggest anything of a practical nature that might avoid those bee stings and lead to fine sweet quince juice for the couple. The most extreme he gets is in this line where he says that some women 'who feel bored by uncompromising and virtuous men and take more pleasure in consorting with those who like dogs and he goats are a combination of licentiousness and sensuality'. Plutarch cites the myth of Pasiphae, who copulated with a bull, as an example, and this time I'm hoping this is a metaphor rather than an outbreak of animal molestation by sexually unsatisfied wives.

We have covered (a lot) how suspicious Greek men were of women and here I'll toss in yet another reason, they believed that women enjoyed sex more than men. The source for this belief came from high up, as high up as you can get, it came from top god Zeus (known as Jupiter to the Romans, his wife Hera they knew as Juno) during a bit of down time in between messing up people's lives, at least according to Roman poet Ovid. 'Jupiter, expansive with wine, set aside his onerous duties, and relaxing, exchanging pleasantries, with Juno, said, "You gain more than we do from the pleasures of love."'[4]

Zeus/Jupiter had certainly had enough liaisons with women to count as a statistically significant sample to form such an opinion. Although as an almighty, all-powerful and not terribly nice king of the gods, it would be a brave woman indeed who didn't put on a performance in bed of truly dramatic proportions to avoid the god's vengeful temper, this might account for Zeus' confidence in the passionate nature of women. However, Hera/Juno denied that women gained the greatest pleasure from sex and refused to countenance her husband's view. How to settle this argument? The obvious solution would be for Zeus and Hera to get it on and then compare notes but neither of them think of this, possibly because Zeus' endless putting it about has put a strain on that part of their relationship, and instead they send for Tiresias because 'he had known Venus both ways'.

How Tiresias came to experience sex as both a male and a female is a tale that Ovid wastes no more than four lines on, which is criminally short.

> Once, with a blow of his stick, he had disturbed two large snakes mating in the green forest, and, marvellous to tell, he was changed from a man to a woman, and lived as such for seven years. In the eighth year he saw the same snakes again and said 'Since there is such power in plaguing you that it changes the giver of a blow to the opposite sex, I will strike you again, now.' He struck the snakes and regained his former shape, and returned to the sex he was born with.[5]

Come on, don't you want to know what Tiresias' first reaction was to suddenly sprouting a pair of lady boobs upon his formally hairy masculine chest? Not to mention the sudden loss of his penis and his entire status which had derived from his very maleness. There's an epic story to be told about Tiresias and the magical gender-transforming snakes that Ovid doesn't tell, because his poem *Metamorphoses* covers from the beginning of creation to the ascension of Julius Caesar, an expanse of time that renders absolutely everyone mentioned by Ovid a bit player in a much bigger story.

Let us reluctantly put our gender-reassigning serpents to one side and return to Zeus and Hera, who are awaiting that big reveal from Tiresias: who enjoys sex more, men or women, or quite possibly snakes given Tiresias' varied life experience? Tiresias was clear in his response; women did. Hera 'was more deeply upset than was justified than the dispute warranted and damned the one who had made the judgement to eternal night'.[6] Hera had struck Tiresias blind for the crime of answering a question honestly based on his/her own experience. Which made Zeus feel kind of bad for summoning Tiresias in the first place, and because a god cannot void the actions of another god, apparently according to Ovid, the best he could do to compensate Tiresias for his wife blinding him was to give him the gift of prophecy.

I'm not sure that counts as adequate compensation for being blinded by the boss's wife, it is likely to be quite a depressing superpower, who wants to see themselves and everyone they know and love ageing towards death or accidentally tumbling into it via some freak accident involving a stubborn donkey and a pair of pruning shears? So it proves for Tiresias later on his life when it he is once again summoned by a king, a mortal one this time, to answer a question. Given the result of his previous summoning, it's not surprising Tiresias is reluctant. 'If I knew the cause of your invitation, yet I've made the mistake of obeying your order! I should not have come.'[7] Tiresias really should have stayed at home in bed because the King of Thebes who has need of his prophetic powers is a certain King Oedipus. It falls to Tiresias to break the news to Oedipus that he has killed his father and married his mother. Perhaps it is fortunate after all that Hera blinded Tiresias, because he's spared the expression on Oedipus' face as he absorbs this information, and he's also spared the sight of Oedipus, having taken a bit of time absorbing this information, gouging out his own eyes. Which proves there's a silver lining to every tale if you look hard enough for it.

That women enjoy sex is mentioned in the medical text known as *The Hippocratic Writings*. 'Once intercourse has begun, she experiences pleasure throughout the whole time,'[8] so the medical boffins declare, ascribing the cause of this pleasure to a irritation of the womb. However, this pleasure for the woman comes to an abrupt halt if her partner should climax first and 'the pleasure experienced by the woman during intercourse is considerably less than the man's, although it lasts longer'.[9] This conclusion, that women enjoy sex less than men, is based I would suggest on the doctor's observations of men and women orgasming. To the observer, a woman's orgasm may appear to last longer but the man's ejection of 'bodily fluid in his case occurs suddenly and as the result of a more violent disturbance than the woman's'.[10] Basically men make more of a performance at their point of ejaculation, so I can fully understand why the Hippocratic doctors concluded that such twisted contortions of expression and strained, strange noises were an indication of a greater experience of pleasure than what they witnessed of the female climax.

Women enjoying sex features also in the raucous plays of Aristophanes, most notably in *Lysistrata*, when the women of Greece go on a sex strike. They find remaining celibate just as difficult as the men and there are several passages that underline how much they enjoy sex with their husbands. 'Anything else, Lysistrata. We'll do anything else you want us to do but… well, better in the fire than out of the bed. Better with the fire than without the cock! That can never do, darling!'[11]

There is a running gag around the women's 'fuck me slippers' that they wear to seduce their husbands, or in this case unbearably tantalise them, and a line about how the war is meaning they aren't getting the sex they want anyhow.

Lysistrata: Tell me, please, all of you: Do you not miss your husband's pricks? Your sons' father? I mean while he's away at war? I know very well that all of you have your husband away at the moment. Not one of them is here with you. Isn't that so?

Caloniki: Mine, in fact, the poor bugger, has been in Thrace for the last five months. Guarding that idiot of a general, Eucrates.

Myrrhini: And mine, seven months at Pylos.

Lampito: And if mine ever manages to steal away for a quickie, they rush over, nab him by the handle and quickly whisk him away back to the front![12]

These are not the Greek women we are used to hearing, or rather not hearing, the silent statues of chasteness. These are women who wait upon their husbands' returns, 'looking pretty, begemmed, beflowered and plastered with make-up, naked under our see-through saffron gowns and wearing our cute little "fuck-me-please" slippers!'[13]

Although another running gag, and it's one that runs throughout Aristophanes, is the type of sex they are having with their husbands. 'What a lot of bum-torn sluts each and every single one of our sex is!'[14] Which is an open gag about Greek love in Athenian society, so engrained is it in their menfolk that anal sex is the norm.

In *The Assembly Women*, with the women of Athens in charge of the city, the men worry what they are going to go with this power.

Blepyrus: Hmmm. I… I fear for us, you know? I fear that for men of our age, when these women take over they'll force us… they'll force us to… well, you know, to…

Chremes: To do what?

Blepyrus: What else? To have sex with them, man! And if we won't be able to do it then we won't even get breakfast!

Chremes: Stupid man! You can do this, can't you? *[Indicates cunnilingus.]* Do it and you'll get both, breakfast and sex!

Blepyrus: But it sure is awful when you're forced to do it.[15]

Clearly Greek men can't be completely oblivious to their women, for they recognise what is the most pleasurable sexual act for women, cunnilingus. Although the joke here is more along the lines of how humiliating this will be for the men because it makes them subservient to their women, which is the crunch joke of the whole play.

Cunnilingus is clearly a favourite subject of Aristophanes because it gets a mention in several of his surviving plays, most notably as an ongoing joke aimed at his rival playwright, Ariphrades, who he credits as having invented the act. 'You mean you haven't heard? Some are born vile, some have vileness thrust upon them but he invented vileness. Thrives on it. Just listen to him play the flute, then think of the whores that mouth has blown. Just imagine that filthy, acrobatic tongue.'[16] References to Ariphrades' bedroom antics also make it into another Aristophanes play *The Wasps*: 'He licked them up every time he went into a brothel,'[17] and pops up in *Peace* as a throwaway line: 'Servant: Who? Ariphrades, he wants her brought his way. Trygaeus: No I can't bear his dirty, sloppy ways.'[18]

From which we might conclude that Aristophanes really did not like Ariphrades and was happy to publicly humiliate him given any opportunity. Publicly being the key word here because Greek comedy plays were enormously popular, they played a huge role in the big festivals of the time such as the Dionysia festival. As part of the festivities, there were competitions for the best plays. Sadly, diddly squat of Ariphrades' output has survived so we have no inkling whether he retaliated in kind for these jibes.

Men, as we have seen, were the dominant force in all aspects of Greek society and the bedroom was no different. Aristophanes' references to Ariphrades as the inventor of cunnilingus is a slur of the worst kind because it makes Ariphrades subservient to a woman, her vagina is penetrating his mouth.

Greek comedy subverts the norm of patriarchy, the women in Aristophanes are very far removed from what our other male authors have told us women were like. These women speak their minds and take world events into their own hands. Politically women never did and never were going to storm the Acropolis and seize power as they do in *The Assembly Women* or be the ones initiating a peace process such as in *Lysistrata*. The premise for both plays is less a critique of women and their foibles but more a very barbed commentary on the Athenian politicians of the day, who Aristophanes dubs so bad that you may as well let women rule because they couldn't make any more of a hash of it.

Practicalities – how to have fun without adding to your food bill

Plato, in creating his ideal society, ponders the biggies of marriage, divorce and death. If a couple should have 'an unfortunate incompatibility of temper',[19] as he puts it, then first those fearsome matrons will decide whether they can be reconciled and if not they may find new partners but only if the marriage has produced no children or an insufficient number of them. If a wife should die without having produced a sufficient number of children, the widowed husband will be compelled to remarry in Platoland until 'he has begotten a sufficient number of sons to his family and the state'.[20] You will have noted Plato's repeated use of 'sufficient'. What was a sufficient number of children for Plato? 'Two children one of either sex, shall deemed sufficient in the eye of the law.'[21]

There is a glaring flaw in Plato's perfectly sized family in his perfectly formed state: how did a couple prevent their sufficient number of children from becoming an abundance? Aristotle, who shared Plato's vision of an ideal state comprised of the right number of children, is brutally clear in how the birth rate should be controlled: 'when couples have an excess of children, let abortion be procured before sense and life have begun.'[22] A pronouncement he spectacularly cops out from taking any responsibility for by adding, 'what may or may not be lawfully done in these cases depends on the question of life and sensation.' Not unlike modern politicians, Aristotle has an idea but he's not volunteering himself to work out the niggly details of that idea.

Compulsory abortion is one of Aristotle's lighter suggestions, certainly compared to this chilling line: 'as to the exposure and rearing of children, let there be a law that no deformed child shall live.'[23] It seems the Spartans weren't alone in feeling fully justified in letting a less than perfect child die. The exposure of babies was widespread in antiquity and accepted as a method of family planning in a matter-of-fact way that is chilling reading for us in the modern day. The child didn't have to be deformed, although gynaecologist Soranus has a whole list of things to check for in your newborn to ensure it is healthy and thus worthy of life, to end up abandoned by its parents and left to die. Daughters were expensive and could not contribute to the household in the same way that sons could, girl babies were therefore more at risk of exposure.

In modern times we have a range of highly effective contraceptives to choose from which have given couples the power to produce what they feel is a sufficient number of children for them. According to the Office of National Statistics, in 2023 British families felt 1.06 children to be sufficient for them. If you are puzzling over that 0.6 of a child, let me add that 44 per cent of families with children have one child, 41 per cent have two children and 15 per cent have three or more children. There are other factors at play in the increasing smaller make-up of British families, which if it gets any lower the Office of National Statistics might start counting pets to keep themselves busy, but effective contraception is certainly key.

Ancient Greece did not have highly effective contraceptives, what it did have was a combination of wrong thinking, wishful thinking and magic to prevent pregnancy. Things that might have worked in preventing pregnancy include the rhythm method, still used today, whereby you time intercourse for the least fertile state of a woman's menstrual cycle, and the withdrawal method, whereby a man removes his penis before ejaculation. Neither method can be considered as effective contraception, the rhythm method even today, with all that we know about fertility and the female body, is only considered 75 per cent effective. The ancient Greeks had less knowledge about how the female body worked, as we have seen, and what was normal and not normal menstruation, added to which regular menstruation is linked to nutrition which may have evaded those at the bottom of the income scale. As for the withdrawal method, its effectiveness is dependent on an iron will from the man, split-second timing and absolutely no juices leaking out before the ba-boom moment. None of these factors can be guaranteed.

Both the rhythm and withdrawal methods appear robustly effective when compared to other forms of contraceptives the Greeks used. If anything is going to kill the mood, it's the woman getting out of the bed immediately post-coitus, aka the ba-boom moment, and performing a series of squats and jumps, sneezing and then downing a cold drink. This is apparently a great way of disrupting any sperm from completing their journey, it's also a sure-fire way of casting suspicion on the soundness of your mind from your perplexed partner. Similar jiggling around is recommended for inducing miscarriages.

White lead was thought to have contraceptive properties if smeared on the vulva, think for a moment on what we know white lead in make-up did to the faces of Tudor women and then wince. Aristotle's contraceptive suggestions are far more benign that white lead, such as myrrh and frankincense. Neither is an effective contraceptive but at least you'll smell nice. Aristotle's Aromas, a missed opportunity if ever I heard one.

Other ingredients of your larder that could be smeared around your lady parts to prevent pregnancy were honey and olive oil, olive oil providing a useful lubricant at the same time, honey not so much. Both of these are preferable to the Egyptian method of using crocodile dung or later Roman suggestions of vulture dung, which harbours at least the potential for being a highly effective contraceptive by repelling any would-be sexual partner from full intercourse when presented with a vulva full of animal poo. Some of these would have been used in pessaries which might have worked as a barrier to the sperm, even if the ingredients used had no effect on the lifespan of sperm.

Outside the realm of medicine, the Magical Papyri contain a spell for preventing pregnancy, which unfortunately we only have in fragments so we cannot test its effectiveness. On the magical amulet side of things, Pliny the Elder, a Roman writer from the first century CE, suggests women wear a part of a lioness's womb in an ivory tube or two worms found in the head of a certain spider. Or you could always pray to your favourite god in advance or afterwards, which contraceptive-wise has the benefit of being convenient, free of charge and likely as effective in preventing pregnancy as most other suggestions from the time.

Sisters are doing it for themselves – sex toys and Sappho

As we've discussed in previous chapters, ancient Greece up to the age of Alexander the Great was a country perpetually at war with itself. These ongoing conflicts took husbands away from their wives for long periods of time and, according to Aristophanes, these lonely women had found an outlet for the resulting frustration: dildos.

It features in *Lysistrata*. 'From the time those Milesians betrayed us, we can't even find our eight-fingered leather dildos. At least they'd serve as a sort of flesh-replacement for our poor cunts.'[24] And: 'I can see the poor love dying to do it the Ionian way a dildo will send her desire away.'[25]

Comedy obviously is not a documentation of a society as it is, otherwise it wouldn't be comedy because let's face it, most of life is mundane and dull. People aren't going to make the effort to leave the house, let alone hand over money for the pleasure of watching two hours of you shovelling handfuls of kettle crisps into your gob whilst watching Saturday-night game shows, entertainment it is not. Comedy takes on a culture and pokes fun at its customs and rituals, often using exaggeration to increase the laughs. It would be easy to throw away the references to dildos that litter the output of Aristophanes as just a joke; however, the key message and indeed target of all Aristophanes' works is the political sphere. He lampoons politicians mercilessly and writers also, not just Ariphrades who we mentioned earlier. Euripides is another writer who is the frequent butt of Aristophanes' gags. In doing so, Aristophanes is documenting the now, he's writing about a real society and including real people that lived in that society.

Aristophanes, as well as documenting the political sphere, is also referencing the private sphere of the society he lived in, there are jokes relating to elite Athenians having all been the passive recipient of anal sex, highlighting the practice of so-called Greek love in Athenian society, and stripping it of its supposedly noble and virtuous purpose for the sake of making a good bum gag. Dildos had to exist somewhere in Aristophanes' world, otherwise nobody would get the joke; for it to work in a non-dildo-owning society he would need a scene in *Lysistrata* of the women making the fake penises.

What also backs up Aristophanes' account of the ancient Greek dildo is that he is not the only writer that mentions them. Herodas was a playwright who lived sometime in the third century BCE, possibly in Alexandria in Egypt, which is about all we know about him. Like Aristophanes he wrote comedies, but the comedies of Herodas are an entirely different genre to Aristophanes' plays because Herodas wrote mimes. Mime in ancient Greece bears no resemblance to modern mime performances: they are not silent and nor are they painfully embarrassing to watch in a way that has you digging your fingernails into your palms until thankfully it is all over. Known in Greek as *mimiamboi*, a combination of the words mine and iambics, mimes were short dramatic scenes which adhered to certain rhythms of words (such as iambic pentameter) and whose plot was geared towards the enjoyment of the common man. Which is a polite way of saying that mimes were populist entertainment that veered strongly towards the coarse.

Certainly, Aristophanes was not shy of using a good knob gag and his plays are, I think we can all agree, coarse. The level of coarseness in Aristophanes depends on which translation you are reading but even the primmest of interpreters can't avoid it entirely. However, Aristophanes' plays, knob and vagina jokes aside, are satirical digs at society and those that run it – there is a point to them as sharp as a pencil brought on the first day of term. I'm not sure the same can be said of mimes, there is no deep political satirising going on underneath the surface, there is no underneath, no depths to explore.

Mime VI of Herodas is usually given the title of 'The Gossiping Friends' or 'An Intimate Chat'. Sometimes it gets given a subtitle of 'The Scarlet Dildo', which I much prefer and will hereafter refer to it as such. 'The Scarlet Dildo' consists of only 100 lines, to put this in context Aristophanes' *Lysistrata* is just shy of 1,300 lines, as is Euripides' tragedy *Electra*, although his satyr play *The Cyclops* is half the length of the rest of his output at around 600 lines, but this is still six times the length of a mime. The shortness of mime as an artform tells us what it was and what it was not, 100 lines is not enough for a fully formed plot with underlying themes of gravitas. However, 100 lines is enough for a comedy skit or sketch, if you like.

'The Scarlet Dildo' is a single scene which I shall have a go at summarising for you. Metro is visiting her friend, Korrito, to ask her whether she can borrow her scarlet dildo. But Korrito has lent it out to many other ladies; however, she does know who made the all-satisfying scarlet dildo. Metro begs Korrito to tell her who made the dildo, Korrito finally divulges it was the cobbler Kerdon. The end.

In between line 1 and line 100 are a series of gags you'll only understand if you know ancient Greek, because they rely on two words sounding similar in that language and a lot of gags you'll only understand if you are ancient

Greek because they rely on knowing that figs are a euphemism for lady parts and that 'keeping chickens' means something terrifically filthy. Any twenty-first-century person thrown amongst an ancient Greek audience watching 'The Scarlet Dildo' is going to find it puzzling experience, like a parent trying to get to grips with emoji language or *Fortnite*. It's just not meant for us.

Much of the hilarity of 'The Scarlet Dildo' may fly straight over our heads, but what is interesting is that in a patriarchal society that very much considered women as 'other', a short skit about two female friends enjoying themselves having a good gossip about how randy they and their friends are should exist at all. Likely it's a pastiche of what men imagine women talk about when they're not around, sex, but I like to believe that Metro and Korrito are based on real women because they seem like a lot of fun.

> Women! That woman will be the death of me one day. I gave in to her pleading and let her have it, Metro, before I had even tried it out myself, but she snatches it up like a door prize and hands it over to women who shouldn't touch it. To hell with her! What a friend! Let her find someone else to pal around with instead of me from now on.[26]

Outside of literature we find images of women using dildos depicted on Greek crockery, this likely falls under the type of crockery to be found at a *symposium* given the titillation factor of a naked lady squatting over an upright dildo or holding one in her hand, looking very much like she's about to perform oral sex on it, as she is penetrated from behind by a man. There's also an intriguing image of a woman climbing into what appears to be a basket of dildos, or the hacked-off penises of men, it's open to interpretation. If it helps with your interpreting, the alternate side of this particular vase depicts the same woman naked, apparently washing herself, we can see a strigil hanging on the wall and her shoes are lined up behind her. So is she cleaning herself up after enjoying the basket full of dildos/severed penises or washing in anticipation of the contents of the basket? There is no answer to this question, I'm afraid, the cataloguers of such images leave their imaginations at home and merely say what they see: 'Erotic, naked woman with phallos climbing into basket with phalloi, stool b: domestic, naked woman at bell krater on block, stool, shoes, sponge and strigil suspended.'[27] A description that in no way does justice to either of the images featured on the vase.

The images depicted of women with dildos appear on crockery very much for the male gaze, one image in particular shows a standing naked women holding up a dildo to her mouth and another dildo in her other hand towards her vagina. What makes this image stand out is how improbable it is, not necessarily the act of double penetration, people are bafflingly (and sometimes disturbingly) diverse in their sexual kinks, but that the woman is performing this double penetration standing up. You'd lie down, really you would, because it is by far the easiest and most comfortable way to achieve this double penetration. So why is she standing up?

Greek vases painters prove themselves competent over and over again in portraying horizontal sex acts, my eyes are glazed over from having trawled through so many, so it is not a question of artistic competence. We discussed in an earlier chapter the nature of the entertainment on offer at a *symposium*, about how prostitutes were often participants, could this be a representation of some of the more risqué entertainments on offer? I think it's a distinct possibility.

The city of Miletus, now in modern-day Turkey, appears to be the dildo capital of the Greek world, it even gets a namecheck in *Lysistrata*. 'And since Milesians went against us,

I've not seen a decent eight-inch dildo.'[28] The note for this line in the translation of *Lysistrata* I am looking at informs me that, 'That city was associated with sexuality and (in this case) the manufacture of sexual toys.'[29] What was manufactured in Miletus is what was known as an *olisbos*. *Olisbos* translates from the ancient Greek as to slide or glide, these sliding/gliding objects were made from stuffed leather and we can presume came in different colours; Aristophanes mentions black and then there's the aforementioned scarlet version. There is a suggestion that olive oil was used as a lubricant.

So we've had references to leather dildos and to scarlet dildos, let me now introduce the *olisbokollikes*, also known as the bread dildo, not so much a bread stick but a bread dick. The joke to end all jokes on the subject of dildos, it's a cracker and I make no apologies for it, This is the perfect place to pause in a chapter titled *Men, Women and Sex* and contemplate how far we've moved away from the men element. Yes, men do feature in some of the images involving dildos and yes, some of the discussion around them is titillation for men, but there has also been an unusual, for ancient Greek society, emphasis on women's enjoyment. In the case of dildos, this was an enjoyment that didn't require the participation of a man, the same is true of our next topic, lesbianism.

Love on Lesbos

Much of our language and understanding of the world has come down to us from the ancient Greeks and, let's face it, by ancient Greeks we mean ancient Greek men. Ancient Greek men are the philosophers, they were the athletes, the doctors and the artists that crafted a civilisation. Ancient Greek women were there but they were at home, generally excluded from public life without a platform for their words, nearly everything we know about ancient Greek women we know because of an ancient Greek man. We see ancient Greek women through the eyes of ancient Greek men; however, and it's a big however, there are exceptions and the biggest exception of them all came from the island of Lesbos.

You'll know the name of this poet, even if you know nothing else about her, which is nothing to be ashamed of because nobody else knows much about her either, even academics who have made her their life's work. Her name was Sappho and she lived on the island of Lesbos in the late seventh/early sixth century BCE. She wrote poetry, of which some 200-odd fragments have survived, and at some point, we can assume she died. That is it, that is all we know about Sappho the living person. Though she lacks much of a biography, Sappho is enormously influential today in her stance as a gay icon, in fact *the* gay icon, for is from her that we get the very word to describe same-sex love between women, lesbian, and the phrase 'sapphic love'.

Despite her obscure origins, Sappho was not picked out of obscurity to represent girl-on-girl action, no, Sappho was enormously famous throughout the centuries that separate her from us. Sappho's reputation in the ancient world was huge and it wasn't centred exclusively around her sexuality, which, let's face it, it tends to be today, but rather on her work and her noted talent.

In Greek mythology, there were nine so-called muses, goddesses who oversaw different aspects of knowledge. There was Clio, who was the muse of history, Calliope, the muse of epic poetry, Erato, the muse of love poetry, Euterpe, the muse of, Melopomene, the muse of tragedy, Polyhymnia, the muse of hymns, Terpsichore, the muse of dance, Thalia, the muse of comedy, and Urania, the muse of astronomy. For Plato, there is someone missing from this lineup of muses. 'Some say there are only nine muses. How careless! Lo Sappho of Lesbos is the tenth!'[30] Praise indeed!

However, Plato is out-praised by serious Solon the Athenian lawmaker who, on hearing his nephew perform a song of Sappho's, begged him to teach him it and, on being questioned why, Solon replied, 'So once I learn it I may die.'[31] Such was the perfection and beauty of Sappho's poetry that to learn it was to realise that life had nothing more to offer you.

The first-century BCE Roman poet, Catullus, was not only inspired in his own compositions by the poetess from Lesbos, he refers to his real-life lover, the very married Claudia Metella, by the name of Lesbia. Such as in this rather beautiful poem: 'Let us live, my Lesbia, let us love, and all the words of the old, and so moral, may they be worth less than nothing to us!'[32] And then, when things had soured between them, 'Caelius, our Lesbia, *that* Lesbia, that Lesbia, Catullus alone loved more than himself, and all of his own, now at crossroads, and down alleyways, jerks off the brave sons of Rome.'[33] Bitter is the word we are all searching for here.

Catullus is being broken hearted and sobbing into the sleeve of his toga in the 60/50s BCE, seven hundred years after Sappho was alive, such is her influence and fame. Although if you really want to measure fame, you can't get bigger than getting your head slapped on a coin. Catullus, despite his personal fame, never got his head slapped on a coin, nor did Plato. Sappho did. Coins with her face on one side and a lyre on the other can be found amongst the 9,000 artefacts within the British Museum's Department of Coins and Medals.

I could go on further about sublimeness of Sappho's poetry, because plenty of ancient and modern authors do, and I could talk more about her stardom, but you're not reading a book entitled *Sex and Sexuality* for literary criticism, presumably, so let's get onto the lesbianism!

In the fragments of Sappho's poetry that have survived, there are many that are about her love and appreciation of girls. 'As for you girls, the gorgeous ones.'[34] There is mention of Arrhis, about whom Sappho declares, 'I loved you once, years ago,'[35] Mnasis, who she'd like to give 'rich gifts which you with your fine cheeks deserve',[36] there is the girl that got away: 'Go with my blessing if you go always remembering what we did,'[37] and then there is the girl who inspires this reaction in Sappho: 'my tongue is shattered. Gauzy flame run radiating under my skin, all that I see is hazy, my ears are all thunder.'[38] Which is perhaps the greatest description ever of how it feels when you really, really fancy someone.

That Sappho fancied, loved and had affairs with girls is written all over her poetry and indisputable, but how typical was she? Were there others like her present in ancient Greece? In other words, where are all the lesbians?

Well, they are certainly not as easy to locate as male lovers. Outside of Sappho, you are hard pressed to find examples of women loving women, mention of the subject is far less copiously mentioned than that of the allegedly morally improving Greek love. Lesbians do get a brief mention in that ode to Greek love, Plato's *Symposium*, where Aristophanes in his speech references women who turn to women.

Women who turn to women were to be found in Sparta too. Plutarch puts this down to the acceptance of same-sex relations between men in Sparta: 'moreover, though this sort of love was so approved among them that even the maidens found lovers in good and noble women',[39] claiming that 'there was no jealous rivalry in it'. Jealous rivalry, perhaps not, but given that Spartan husbands were encouraged to spend as little time with their wives as possible, we might see this as a release from sexual frustrations and generally unsatisfactory Spartan men. Spartan women's dissatisfaction with their menfolk is detailed at length in Plutarch's collated *Sayings of Spartan Women* where they appear largely indifferent to the death of any of their menfolk. Take this example: 'Gyrtias, when on a time Acrotatus, her grandson, in a fight with other boys received many blows, and was brought home for dead, and the family and friends were all wailing, said, "Will you not stop your noise? He has shown from what blood he was sprung."'[40] In an atmosphere of such disdain for men if they should stray even slightly from the Spartan ideal, it is perhaps not surprising the Spartan women turned to each other, there was less disappointment to be had.

Another place you do find mentioned women loving women is in spells. Magic spells are very popular in antiquity as a way of dealing with the day-to-day problems of life, such as how to win dice games – 'Into your hand say: "Let not even one person be equal to me, for I am THERTHENITH-R

ER-THORTHIN DOLMHOR, and I am going to throw what I want." And say this repeatedly, and then throw'[41] – how to introduce insomnia in other people, gaining favour and friendship forever (centuries before *How to Make Friends and Influence People* was published), and how to keep bugs out of your house. The last of which requires access to a goat: 'Mix goat bile with water and sprinkle it. To keep fleas out of the house: Wet rosebay with salt water, grind it and spread it.'[42] Practical, every day, useful spells that we could all do with.

Love spells were particularly prized and it is amongst these that we find a spell written in Greek that was discovered in Egypt. In this spell, Herais begs the Egyptian god Anubis and the Greek god Hermes to 'attract and bind Sarapias, whom Helen bore, to this Herais, whom Thermoutharin bore, now, now; quickly, quickly. By her soul and heart attract Sarapias herself, whom Helen bore from her own womb.'[43]

Another spell from the third/fourth century and found in what was the Greek city of Hermopolis and what is now part of Egypt, mentions two women, Sophia and Gorgonia: 'Inflame the heart, the liver, the spirit of Gorgonia, whom Nilogenia bore, with love and affection for Sophia.'[44]

This is a fairly meagre selection of lesbians, which, given the patriarchal nature of the Greek city states and the empires that later swallowed them up such as the Macedonians and Romans, is hardly surprising. But it's interesting that one of the few genuine female voices from antiquity we have, Sappho, is so very open and unashamed of her love for women. Perhaps if we had access to more female voices we might discover the same, after all, Greek husbands were frequently away from home fighting or courting boys to inspire, the women had time to fill…

Chapter 15

Rape and Sexual Assault

There was no escaping the subject of rape in ancient Greece, it was woven into the fabric of their society. Greek religion abounds with stories of rape or attempted rape ranging from the troubling to the downright disturbing.

Olympian rules

From the Trojan War we have Cassandra, a princess of Troy, who, as her city was being destroyed around her by the Greeks, took sanctuary in the temple of Athena where she should have been safe. She wasn't. Ajax burst in and raped her within the goddess's sanctuary. Later she is handed over to the leader of the Greek forces, Agamemnon, as one of the spoils of war to be taken back with him to Mycene. The 'hero' Achilles has his own spoil of war, Briseis, who is his slave and the cause of an argument with his commander, Agamemnon, who demands he hand her over to him, which Achilles does. And what about Helen, the Queen of Sparta, who started off this war? In some versions of the myth, she is Paris' willing lover and departs freely with him, in others she is forcibly taken by Paris because the goddess Aphrodite had promised her to him.

From the above, it should be clear now that the word 'hero' had a very different meaning in ancient Greece compared to how we deploy it today. We like our heroes to be inspirational, admirable and flawless. We require them to be as close to perfection as possible and any that fail to live up to our esteem are quickly cut down by the tabloid press, at least they are in the UK. Greek heroes had flaws, whopping chasms of flaws that sealed their destiny and their fate, that fate was likely no happy ending. They were not there to inspire the ordinary Greek to greatness or to be held up as examples for small children to emulate, instead they served as a warning as to the dark places the flaws of man could lead him.

King Agamemnon looms large in Greek mythology as a great warrior and victor of the Trojan War, but he was not a man to be admired. He sacrificed his own daughter, Iphigenia, to please the goddess Artemis into helping them sail to Troy.

Sacrifice is another word that we use differently today, we might casually sacrifice lunch in anticipation of a large dinner or sacrifice our time for a good deed. The sacrifice of Iphigenia falls under the second distinctly unpleasant definition of the word: 'Sacrifice: to kill an animal or person and offer them to a god or gods.'[1] Although in some versions of the story Iphigenia escapes her father's attempts to murder her, perhaps because it was too horrible an ending even for the ancient Greeks.

All of the heroes I have namechecked in this chapter come to sticky ends. Achilles dies during the battle for Troy, shot by an arrow that penetrates his sole point of weakness, his ankle. Agamemnon is hacked to death in the bath by his wife Clytemnestra, furious at what he had done to their daughter and for arriving home with his new sex toy, Cassandra. Ajax's end varies in its telling, but in most tales he loses his mind and commits suicide. So much for the heroes of Troy.

Although the gods may have played a role in the downfall of the victors of Troy, they were no better behaved when it comes to the topic of sexual assault. Although their actions tend to have less consequences, if any, for the divine. The nymph Daphne was so desperate to escape the enforced clutches of the god Apollo that she was turned into a laurel tree, an event beautifully captured in marble by seventeenth-century sculptor Bernini. Bernini also portrayed in stone another god-on-goddess rape, that of Persephone by Hades, god of the underworld. Both of Bernini's sculptures, one depicting an attempted rape and the other a successful rape attempt, are housed in the Borghese Gallery in Rome and rate as two of the most accomplished, mind-blowingly mesmerising, beautiful and greatest works of art in all of art history. Which is troubling to the viewer, given the very unbeautiful and dark acts they depict.

The attempted rape of Daphne would gift the world an additional laurel tree, the rape of Persephone would have much bigger implications for mankind. Persephone was the daughter of Demeter, the goddess of agriculture, grain, bread and all the bounty the earth had to offer mankind. With Hades having taken her daughter with him to his underground kingdom, Demeter mourned. She spent her days desperately searching for her beloved child and neglecting her goddess duties. This was a big deal given what she was goddess of.

I mean, we could probably all get by if, say, Iris, goddess of the rainbow, took a week's holiday. Rainbows are pretty and colourful and all that, but I suspect you can't remember in any detail the last time you saw one. Similarly, it might be nice if Nemesis, the goddess of vengeance and retribution, took a gap year abroad, giving mankind a break from all those negative feelings boiling up inside us. Yes, I'm looking at you, Hesiod, and that barn-stealing hussy you can't forgive. But Demeter was a top-drawer goddess, one of the twelve key Olympian deities entrusted with the huge responsibility of providing the very food on our tables.

So key is Demeter that Hesiod includes prayers to her as part of his essential guide to being a farmer in bloody awful times: 'Pray to Zeus of the earth and to pure Demeter to make Demeter's holy grain sound, and heavy when first you begin ploughing.'[2] There is in Hesiod's mind a payoff for this venerating of the goddess: 'venerable Demeter richly crowned may love you and fill your barn with food.'[3] With the added warning to his fellow farmers: 'both gods and men are angry with a man who lives idle.' Although I suspect for the idle farmer Hesiod is probably the greater threat, and likely to be the one slagging him off to the neighbours whilst offering prayers up to Demeter that his harvest fails and he starves to death.

With Demeter otherwise engaged, the earth was not bountiful, it was barren and a barren earth meant famine for those living on it. This was disastrous, so disastrous that Zeus intervened, which is quite something because in most myths Zeus seems quite happy to let mankind suffer and indeed is often the cause of that suffering. Remember the story of how Zeus inflicted toil and illness on all of mankind who had never known either because Prometheus had shown them his fire trick?

But Zeus does intervene in this case, perhaps because if Demeter succeeds in killing everyone off in a mass famine he'll have no little men to play cruel games with and little women to abduct and impregnate. Another mitigating factor in Zeus' intervention might be due to Persephone being his daughter, and also his niece, because Demeter happens to be his sister, which is the way Greek myths tend to go. Zeus' missus, the Queen of Olympia, Hera, is another of his sisters. His other sister, Hestia, goddess of the hearth/fire, is spared Zeus' sexual attentions, you'll be glad to hear, although her brother Poseidon and her nephew Apollo both attempt to woo her and both fail. Hestia is allowed by her biggest, meanest brother Zeus to maintain her virginity. It's fair to say that as a family the Olympian gods are messed up beyond the wildest soap opera writer's imagination.

So Persephone, because of Zeus' power over the other gods (did I mention that Hades is Zeus and Demeter's brother, making him Persephone's uncle?), is returned to her mother, sort of. Because whilst being in the underworld she had fatefully eaten some pomegranate seeds that meant she could never fully leave Hades' kingdom. A compromise was reached whereby Persephone would spend half the year with Hades as his queen and half the year with her mother. It was a compromise Demeter was not prepared to accept and she mourned every month her daughter was missing, which for ancient Greeks explained away why crops do not grow in winter but food became bountiful in the spring and summer when Persephone was allowed to visit her mum.

Bernini's statue, mentioned earlier, captures the moment of Persephone's abduction by her uncle, such is the artist's skill that you can see Hades' fingers digging into the soft flesh of her upper thigh. Bernini was not the first artist to depict mythological rape in art, you will find sexual assault reproduced in a myriad of paintings and sculptures scattered across the great museums of the world. You've no doubt walked past them without a second thought or maybe clocked the title and its use of words such as 'abduction' and 'seduction', which sanitise and lessen the act being committed.

Rape was a big feature of ancient Greek art too, depictions of gods assaulting mortal women are to be seen frequently on Greek vases, which to our modern eyes is a very inappropriate topic to feature on a breakfast bowl or wine cooler.

An accepted part of life?

The sheer number of stories from Greek mythology that involve rapes, most of which have no consequences for – or even enhance the rank of – the rapist, such as Hades, whose victim becomes his ruling queen, might lead us to conclude that rape was generally tolerated in Greek society. This is also borne out by its appearance as a plot line in numerous comedies.

The Arbitration by third-century BCE comic playwright, Meander, features as its plotline (in the 750 lines of it that have survived) Pamphile and Charisios, whose marriage is blown apart by Pamphile giving birth to a child that could not possibly be her husband's as it occurred only five months after their wedding. Charisios being away on business at the time of the birth, a desperate Pamphile abandons the child, but crucially she drapes the baby in some of her jewellery, which will prove to be very important to the plot later on. When Charisios returns, one of the slaves lets him on the secret and he walks out on Pamphile, spending his days drinking away her dowry and taking up with a prostitute.

Meanwhile, Pamphile's abandoned baby is picked up by a passing shepherd who intends to keep the jewels for himself. A legal argument follows as to whether the jewels belong to the shepherd or the baby. A ruling is made that they belong to the baby when the judge recognises the jewellery and thus the identity of the child.

Elsewhere, Charisios is beginning to tire of his good life and miss his wife, especially when he overhears that she is thinking of divorcing him. Cue a happy ending Greek style when Charisios' prostitute lover improbably enters, holding the baby, and reveals to Pamphile that she knows who the father of the baby is, it's Charisios himself! So everything is fine, and the couple can reunite and form a happy family with their child. If you're wondering how neither Pamphile nor Charisios know that he is the father of the child, it's because Pamphile had been raped at a festival by an unknown assailant, that unknown assailant being her own husband. So that's all okay then, woman lives happily ever after with the type of husband who doesn't even stop to check the identity of the woman he is raping at a local festival.

This plot again underlines how much rape is a crime against men, there is no dishonour for Charisios for being a rapist because he hasn't raped the wife of another man, dishonouring and bringing shame to that *oikos*. No, the happy reveal for the couple is that Pamphile was sexually assaulted by her husband.

A remarkably similar plot is to be found in another of Meander's plays, *The Woman from Samos*. This time, Moschion must admit it is he who raped his intended bride, Plangon, and is thus the father of her illegitimate child, before they can happily proceed with the wedding. Although Moschion isn't entirely off the hook, the chorus at least throw a bit of judgement his way:

> And even though he does love Plangon and wants to marry her, he's forgotten that he did assault her and have a child out of wedlock with her – which is a very serious deal … If a girl's father found out that his daughter had been assaulted and raped by some rich little punk, he had the right to make a public example of him by taking a large radish – or they had a certain species of fish, the mullet, which had spikes sticking out of its head – and he would insert it into the offender's posterior – not a punishment for Moschion to take sitting down. In fact, it'd be while before he did any type of sitting, I'd guess.[4]

Moschion does not get a fish stuffed up his arse, more's the pity, he ends up marrying his bride/victim. Elsewhere in Aristophanes' *The Acharnians*, Dicaeopolis fantasises about raping a slave: 'O Phales, dear Phales, what bliss if I could creep up on Thratta, that beautiful maid, Strymodorus's girl, who works in his wood, as she's stealing boughs from a Phelleus glade. I'd grab her two arms, throw her down double quick, and harvest her cherry with my throbbing prick.'[5]

That a man violating a woman at a festival or fantasising about forcing himself upon a slave girl is served up as something to laugh at and that both men and women attended festivals and worshipped gods who routinely violated mortal women sexually suggests that rape wasn't taken as seriously as an offence in ancient Greece as it is today. The cultural gap between how the ancient Greeks viewed rape compared to our twenty-first-century society is even bigger than this: in ancient Greek there is no word for rape.

Sex is sex

The dictionary definition of the word rape in English is to 'force someone to have sex when they are unwilling, using violence or threatening behaviour'.[6] Under the Sexual Offences Act 2003, a perpetrator found guilty of the intentional penetration of a vagina, anus or mouth without consent, or when the perpetrator does not reasonably believe they have consent, could be imprisoned for life. In ancient Athens, there was no criminal offence of rape, that is being penetrated sexually without your consent, the offence occurred if there was violence involved, where it was treated the same as getting roughed up in the street after a particularly wine-heavy *symposium*. That an attack upon a person might feature a sexual assault was irrelevant to the charge, the ancient Greeks did not have a word for nor share the understanding we do today regarding rape.

Today we recognise rape as a crime inflicted upon women; although men can obviously be raped too, the overwhelming majority of victims are women. We see mass rapes of women used as deliberate tactic during conflicts in places like Sierra Leone and Bosnia. The terrorist group Isis captured girls during its bloody rampage across the Middle East and sold them as sex slaves openly in markets. In Britain, women from poorer countries are tricked into entering the country by gangs and forced into prostitution. Even British citizens, young girls from across the UK, have been targeted by grooming gangs and forced into having sex with multiple men a night.

Rape is very much a crime perpetrated against women by men, often under the influence of a malignant misogyny and rage. In ancient Greek times, it was considered a crime against the victim's husband or other male relatives. If you think that is shocking, let me lob another hand grenade to blow your mind: in ancient Greece, adultery, that is having consensual sex with a woman who was married to another man, was considered a greater crime than forcing yourself upon a woman married to another man.

We saw this in the murder trial we featured in a previous chapter where the seduction of the wife of Euphiletos was centre stage in the case, with the murder itself barely having a light shone on it. This is because the real crime is not the murder of Eratosthenes but the victim's own actions towards the defendant's wife. As Euphiletos says in his defence:

> The assumption is that those who achieve their aims by force are hated by those they have violated, while seducers so corrupt the souls of their victims that they make other men's wives more intimate with them than they are with their husbands. They make the whole house theirs, and it becomes unclear to which father the children belong, the husband or the seducer. Because of this the lawmaker assigned death as the penalty for seducers.[7]

Again, this demonstrates the Greek male paranoia about women that we saw with the likes of Hesiod, as well as demonstrating the importance of the *oikos* in Greek society. The penetration of the *oikos* by this interloper 'brought shame on my children and insulted me by entering my house'.[8] Euphiletos' responsibilities as head of the *oikos* are towards the preservation of his family's wealth, reputation and taking care of the individual members of the *oikos*, particularly the womenfolk. He has failed on all scores.

We talked a bit about why Greek men were so paranoid about women in earlier chapters based on the fear that a bad wife might be wasteful of a husband's hard work, but it is worth revisiting it in this context. A man was tasked with preserving the *oikos* that had been built up by his ancestors, women were brought into it as strangers who didn't have the same attachment to this heritage, indeed on divorce or death a woman might find herself moving into the *oikos* of another man. The *oikos* was permanent, women were transient yet also held the power to damage that which they left behind.

Whether Euphiletos got off his murder charge or not (we don't know the outcome of his trial), his household was damaged goods. His wife, or rather ex-wife, the law demanding that Euphiletos divorce her, walked away from the *oikos*, leaving it tainted with shame. She might have, though she didn't, have left a further bundle of shame behind in the shape of a child that was not her husband's, thus destroying the bloodline of the *oikos*, the ultimate shame for a Greek man. Which in some ways again explains their paranoia of women, the many ways in which they sought to control women's behaviour because their actions, or even actions that happened to them, such as rape, impacted the *oikos*, so integral to the Greek man's authority and reputation in the city amongst his peers.

Could a man who took so little care of his household that an intruder raped his wife, or failed to notice another man was seducing his wife under his very nose, be trusted? Should such a man be entrusted with public office, was such a man useful by your side in battle? At a bare minimum his judgement was suspect. Gossip mattered in ancient Athens, it held the power to disrupt your public life whilst your private life exploded all around you.

The law

Although there is no word for rape, as we understand it, sex that was not part of a seduction does feature as prosecutable. In Athens, in a law laid down by Solon, 'he permitted an adulterer caught in the act to be killed; but if a man committed rape upon a free woman, he was merely to be fined a hundred drachmas'.[9] A ruling that Solon's first-century-CE-dwelling biographer considers 'very absurd'. Not included in this ruling were 'those who sell themselves openly, meaning of course the courtesans'.[10] A prostitute legally could not be raped, something we shall look into more detail in the next chapter; also exempt from rape laws were slaves.

In fifth-century BCE Crete, in the city state of Gortyn, rape (again the ancient Greek understanding of rape, e.g. sex not as part of an ongoing affair) is also punishable by a fine. How much of a fine is determined by the social class of the woman violated – raping a free woman incurred a fine of 100 staters, whereas for raping a serf the fine was five drachma and 'If one debauch a female house-slave by force he shall pay two staters.'[11]

With a similar attention to the miniscule details, the fines incurred for committing adultery in Gortyn depend not on social class but rather where this adultery took place. If it was in her brother's, father's or husband's house you faced the highest penalty of 100 staters (the same fine, you'll note, for raping a free woman) but if this adultery takes place in the home of another, the fine was a lesser 50 staters.

The prosecutions that come under these laws are brought by men against other men for injury done to the property of men.

The women's tale

We have little evidence for any actual prosecutions for rape but then a rape prosecution was not to the benefit of the violated woman, she was not the victim of the crime, her menfolk were. With no distinction in law between forced and consensual sex, the raped woman could be considered a perpetrator, alongside her rapist, of bringing shame and dishonour to the *oikos*, this created legal consequences for her.

The law in Athens insisted that a woman who had partaken in sex outside of her marriage whichever way it had occurred, whether by consent or not, be divorced from her husband, barred from wearing jewellery and partaking in public ceremonies. Effectively she was a social outcast, unlikely to attract another husband to support her and with no recourse in law to defend herself without the backing of her male guardian, and how many of those were prepared to have their family's shame repeated in public? It's really not surprising that we find some bleak reactions from ancient Greek rape victims.

'Some say that Mycerinus passionately desired his own daughter and then he had intercourse with her against her will. They then say the girl hanged herself in her distress.'[12] And 'because the assault seemed unbearable to the girls they immediately hanged themselves'.[13]

How to marry the distress of these girls with rape as a standard comedy plotline? I don't think we can, and I don't think the ancient Greeks could either as they tumbled between downplaying forced sex as just one of those things, whilst simultaneously worrying how it affected them; putting men and their feelings right at the heart of Greek society. Greek women, in contrast, are rendered bystanders to their own assaults, their bodies, their hurt was irrelevant. It was the hurt and shame caused by their assaults that was important, and only when it affected men.

Chapter 16
Prostitution

Prostitution is sometimes referred to as the world's oldest profession and not without good reason for there is evidence for its existence throughout history. Ancient Greece was no exception, but it was exceptional in how prostitution was regarded compared to our society. In twenty-first-century Britain, technically it isn't illegal to exchange sexual favours for money, but the law makes it damn difficult for you to do so. It is illegal to tout for clients on the street or any other public place, it is illegal to own or manage a brothel, it is illegal to work as a pimp collecting money on behalf of sex workers and it is illegal to advertise sexual services.[1]

All these laws are there to discourage prostitution and work to underline the undesirable nature of sex work by heaping so many restrictions on its practices. Largely these laws have produced the desired effect, prostitution is not an occupation that anyone would openly admit to having, nor is it a service that most men would openly admit to using. Obviously, prostitution is still a feature of twenty-first-century society, but it's not something that is discussed openly, it is taboo, considered shameful and hidden away.

Meanwhile, in ancient Athens, Solon our lawmaking poet from a few chapters ago is being uniformly praised for opening Athens' first brothel. 'O Solon you are our benefactor as our city is full of young men of ardent temperament who could be carried away to punishable acts. But you brought women and installed them in particular places where they can be at disposal of all who need them … Anybody can enjoy them easily without risk day or night.'[2]

It is difficult to imagine any political party in the twenty-first century including in their manifesto a promise to unburden the sexual frustration of young men by setting up government-sponsored brothels. I suppose it might gain them the incel vote, provided they survived a tabloid explosion of moral indignation so forceful as to leave the entire voting population with permanent tinnitus.

Solon himself presented this as a moral law, the moral concern being that without an outlet for their urges the youth of Athens would fall into affairs with married women. This neatly highlights two sections of Athenian society we have touched on previously: women and youths, both of whom are prone to fall into immorality if not given proper guidance from an Athenian man. In this instance, youths were to be guided away from their wives and daughters whose reputation they could destroy (not to mention the humiliation poured all over the husband for being cuckolded by a randy teenager) and guided towards Solon's state-sponsored brothel.

It was a winning scheme; Solon's brothel was so successful that he used the taxes raised from its activities to build a temple to Aphrodite. Which is fitting, I guess. This tax, known as *pornikon teles*, was paid by all prostitutes in Athens. The Greek word for prostitute is *porne*, which is, yes, another gift to the English language from the Greeks because *porne* becomes our pornography.

For those in Solon's brothel, the tax was paid by the manager, prostitutes who worked for themselves had to cough up the money individually. The tax was proportion of their earnings, earnings which surprisingly were set by state and an official known as agoranomos. With prostitution in Athens being both sponsored and encouraged by the state, it is unsurprising that it flourished. It was said that no city had more women working as prostitutes than Athens. A fact that hadn't gone unnoticed by serious philosopher type, Socrates. 'You don't suppose that that lust provokes men to beget children when the streets and stews are full of the means to satisfy that.'[3] To date, archaeologists have identified only one brothel in the ancient city, which doesn't mean they weren't there but maybe just more discreet and subtle than their Roman counterparts.[4]

Prostitution was not an occupation considered suitable for the Athenian citizen. One of Solon's laws was to prohibit men from selling their daughters or sisters to a brothel keeper should the family hit dire straits or to act as their pimp to raise funds themselves. That it was thought necessarily to have this written down in law suggests that it was a situation that some of Athens' female citizens had horrifyingly found themselves trapped in. There was a stinker of a caveat to this seemingly protective law, the abusive family member was subject to prosecution 'unless he finds out she is no longer a virgin'.[8] In which case she has no honour to be protected and can be pimped out to whomever.

For the love of the goddess

Rivalling Athens for the sex worker capital of Greece was Corinth. Corinth was a port city on the Peloponnesian coast and host to the Isthmus Games, which were part of the prestigious Panhellenic Games. It was thus a bustling city and here, according to first-century CE geographer Strabo, there were to be found 1,000 prostitutes working in the sanctuary of Aphrodite. So famous were these prostitutes of Aphrodite that 'the city was crowded with people and grew rich; for instance, the ship captains freely squandered their money, and hence the proverb, "Not for every man is the voyage to Corinth."'[5]

Strabo's description of these Corinthian prostitutes has led to a great deal of scholarly suggestions that this was a form of sacred prostitution, that is sex as a rite or ritual in veneration of a god or goddess. What is important to note up front is that Strabo is not describing anything he witnessed in the first century CE during his own travels, but rather he's reporting back a story from Corinth's past and it's an exaggerated version. We know it's exaggerated because excavations of the Temple of Aphrodite have revealed a much smaller structure than expected, much too small to house 1,000 prostitutes.

Strabo also doesn't mention anything about any accompanying rituals, prayers or sacrifices associated with the prostitutes. The only religious connection he makes is how the prostitutes came to be there; they were votive offerings to the goddess, slaves in other words. These slaves no doubt helped with the upkeep of the sanctuary via the profession they'd been dedicated into.

Remember our efficient tour guide Pausanias who listed all the many, many statues at Olympia? He also set foot in Corinth and he also mentions the Temple of Aphrodite that stands there; however, he makes no mention of prostitution, sacred or otherwise. Thorough compiler of details that he is, I kind of think if sacred prostitution had been a thing in Corinth at any part of their history, then Pausanias would have included it as a titbit for his readers. It's a very titbit-worthy tale, that he doesn't mention it at all is telling, or rather not telling.

Another traveller who clearly found the city of Corinth a little spicy was a chap by the name of Saul of Tarsus. Saul was travelling to Damascus to find some Christians to persecute when,

> suddenly a light from heaven flashed around him. He fell to the ground and heard a voice say to him, 'Saul, Saul, why do you persecute me?' 'Who are you, Lord?' Saul asked.
>
> 'I am Jesus, whom you are persecuting,' he replied. 'Now get up and go into the city, and you will be told what you must do.'[6]

Quicker than you can say 'do you want an ice pack for that lump on your head?' Saul was on his feet ready to fulfil this command/concussion depending on your religious viewpoint. Only when Saul opened his eyes he could see nothing, he was totally blind, which again could either be down to the justifiable annoyance of Jesus for Saul's Christian-persecuting ways or the result of the sort of head injury incurred when you fall off your horse and thump on the road unexpectedly. Saul spent three days blind, neither eating nor drinking, instead he did a lot of thinking, because there was bugger all else he could do, what with being blind and all.

One miraculous unblinding later, Saul was a new man with a new name, Paul, and a new cause to throw himself behind. No longer was he going to spend his energies persecuting Christians, no, he was instead going to spread the word of Christianity for he was now a true believer! Whatever was at the bottom of Saul's abrupt change of personality, you can't fault him for his energy, for he sets himself off to convert as many people, as many cities as he can to the Christian cause.

One such city on Paul's itinerary of inspiration was Corinth and having sorted that out, off he rode into the sunset to the next city that needed his help, a lonesome warrior of words and ideas. Only the Corinthian Christian church he left behind him has not performed as expected, they seem to have missed some major tenets of Paul and Christ's teaching. Hence the very cross letter that Paul writes to them.

> By his power God raised the Lord from the dead, and he will raise us also. Do you not know that your bodies are members of Christ himself? Shall I then take the members of Christ and unite them with a prostitute? Never!

> Do you not know that he who unites himself with a prostitute is one with her in body? For it is said, 'The two will become one flesh. But whoever is united with the Lord is one with him in spirit. Flee from sexual immorality.'[7]

Those famous prostitutes of Corinth are clearly too much for even the devout to resist.

Different types of prostitution

Many books on ancient Greek sexuality seek to neatly categorise sex workers into distinct types, they are aided in this categorisation by the multitude of words that Greeks used to describe prostitutes. As mentioned earlier, *porne* was a blanket term which translates to whore, but under that umbrella term we find words like *katakleista*, meaning 'shut in' and referring to brothel workers. *Chamaitype*, which translates to lie down, these prostitutes worked outdoors in comparison with *perepatetiake*, who wandered the streets picking up men and taking them back to a room. *Gephyriade* plied their trade midway between these two extremes, picking up their trade by bridges and other public monuments. And then there were the most famous of all prostitutes, the high-class, high-end and high-priced *hetairae*.

High class?

Hetaira: the word translates as companion, which can be misleading. As can modern attempts to equate the *hetairae* to the Geisha of Japan, the *hetairae* are a distinct grouping of their own and very much linked to the time and place in which they appear. As we've previously discussed, the ideal Athenian woman stayed at home and same-sex relations were bound to very strict social conventions on both sides. This created a problem for your male Athenian, because after a full day spent hanging out with your best beardy pals at the gym, then at the philosophy school and again at the theatre, well, come the evening you want to mix it up a little. At the very least you want some new gossip that isn't Medes' tall tale about the time he went bull leaping in Crete because you've heard that bollocks three times already that day. Enter the *hetairae*.

The *hetairae* are at the high end of prostitution and they charge far more than an obol. Far more. That it is a *hetaira* who is the plus one for your average Athenian male to take with him to the most fashionable dinner party of the evening is another zinger in our ever-growing list of ways in which the ancient Greeks are really not like us. It is a rare wife indeed in the twenty-first century who would put up with her husband taking a prostitute out to a swanky dinner party instead of her. You would hope that he'd at least bring a doggie bag home for the missus, but I bet he didn't.

Why was a prostitute considered a better dinner party companion than a wife? I keep saying dinner party when what I mean is a *symposium*. You may remember that, according to the author of *Love, Sex and Marriage in Ancient Greece*, 'very often, if not always, the symposium wound up in an orgy'.[9] So, not the kind of place you would want to take your respectable wife to.

The *hetairae* played a number of roles at the *symposium* and indeed instruments. When I say instruments, I mean that they were often proficient in playing the harp and flute to entertain guests. But yes, there was a certain other instrument, less woodwind, more flesh, that they also blew to entertain guests. But what a *hetaira* had that your prostitute selling quickies under an arch did not was conversation. One of the key reasons *hetairae* were the partner of choice to accompany men was that they were known for their witty conversation and keen knowledge, something that Greek wives and daughters were expressly told not to do. Good wives were silent, they did not do conversation, witty or otherwise.

Clearly having someone you could talk to about the matters of the day as an equal was attractive because a number of high-profile, famous types pick a *heterae* to be their long-term partner. The most famous of these was Aspasia.

Aspasia – the hero's whore

'Aspasia, as some say was held in high favour by Pericles because of her rare political wisdom.'[10] So says Pericles' biographer, Plutarch, who then goes onto claim that even Socrates had need of her wisdom and frequently visited her with his disciples. From which we may gather she was a pretty influential woman.

Aspasia, according to Plutarch, was Milesian by birth. Miletus was a city founded by Greek colonists in what is now Turkey. Plutarch's account makes it sound as if Aspasia chose her profession. 'They say that it was in emulation of Thargelia, an Ionian woman of ancient times, that she made her onslaughts upon the most influential men. This Thargelia came to be a great beauty and was endowed with grace of manners as well as clever wits.'[11] We cannot know the truth of it but it's interesting to compare Aspasia's prostitute origins with the story of another prostitute, Neaera, which we shall look at shorty.

Plutarch, writing centuries later about Aspasia, wishes 'to raise the query what great art or power this woman had, that she managed as she pleased the foremost men of the state, and afforded the philosophers occasion to discuss her in exalted terms and at great length'.[12] It's not a query he finds an answer to, but it fascinates him that Socrates seeks her opinion, 'although she presided over a business that was anything but honest or even reputable, since she kept a house of young courtesans'.[13]

He's even more flabbergasted that 'Lysicles the sheep-dealer, a man of low birth and nature, came to be the first man at Athens by living with Aspasia after the death of Pericles'.[14]

Statesman of the era, Pericles, is so taken by her that he found another man for his wife so he could take up with Aspasia as his permanent companion. At which point I like to think Plutarch and I are thinking the same thing: she had to be fabulous in bed. For why else would so many clever men risk their reputations through consulting a lowly prostitute, repeatedly? I am sceptical it was purely for the great political insight she was said to possesses, she was trained in pleasing men and please men she did.

It couldn't last because nobody held onto intellectual or political supremacy in ancient Athens for long, those who flew close to the sun, such as Alcibiades and Socrates, soon had the wings melted off their backs and plummeted out of favour towards a hard and unforgiving world. Such was the story of Aspasia too. Her influence on Pericles had her as well as him blamed for policy failings and she was faced with a malicious trial for committing impiety. Plutarch notes that in the comedies of his day Aspasia is openly referred to as a prostitute, quoting directly from one: 'As his Hera, Aspasia was born, the child of Unnatural Lust, A prostitute past shaming.'[15]

The evidence of the pots

There are various sources that give us an insight into the life of a *hetaira* including literary sources, but one of the richest is Greek red and black pottery. At this point you may be waggling your finger at this book and on the poise of spitting out a 'But!' Yes, I know what I said in a previous chapter about the perils of using images on pottery to make sweeping statements about Greek culture, but pottery really does offer us a valuable insight into *hetairae* and their position in Greek society. If we decide that the extreme sexual images we find on Greek pottery are not an accurate representation of reality then that makes them even more disturbing, because it means they are a representation of what Greek men thought reality should be. A masturbatory fantasy, if you will, one which was not kept behind a bedroom door with the curtains closed but rather shared with your mates and passed around in public at the gym or at a *symposium*.

The *symposium* had its own special kind of cup; known as a kylix, it had two handles and a short stem, and was partly responsible for the insane levels of drunkenness that such events reached. Keeping to the spirit of the evening, kylix cups are the receptacles of the most singularly filthy images you are ever likely to see depicted in antiquity, or indeed any other era.

A quick scan through the list of kylix cups currently housed in the British Museum uncovers such classic scenes as a satyr trying to bonk deer, a naked woman crouched with a dildo in each hand, and 'naked *hetaira* stands on the right and slowly eases herself backwards and downwards onto the man's erect penis, one hand resting on his ribs, the other on his hip, steadying her progress.'[16] That last one I'm quoting directly from the catalogue. Elsewhere we find Wikimedia Commons going coy and sparse when describing a very involved and detailed scene as 'sexual orgy between 5 satyrs'.[17] A summary that loses all the glorious details from this particular cup.

Hetairae feature on a number of such pieces of *symposium* crockery, sometimes they are fully clothed and entertaining the guests with their music or dancing. Sometimes the *hetaira* is depicted naked and being penetrated, usually from behind, by a male. Sometimes they are being penetrated by several men, orally and certainly vaginally and maybe anally as well. Why are so many *hetairae* shown to be penetrated from behind? Was doggy style simply a favourite sexual position of the ancient Greeks? Distressingly, scholars think it is more likely depicted because being taken from behind was seen as humiliating for the recipient. It's hard to see being penetrated by several men at once as anything less than degrading for the woman involved. In our society, such scenes are not to be found in the arthouse erotically charged film genre, they are to be found in cheap, nasty pornography films.

As we've said previously, and repeatedly, these are not necessarily scenes taken from real life, but even if they are entirely fictitious, it tells us something, doesn't it? It tells us that Athenian men desired to humiliate and degrade these supposedly high-class courtesans. Greek men also desired to physically hurt *hetairae*, it would appear from what we find depicted on pottery. There is a running motif of a single sandal found in images, sometimes it is hanging on the wall, acting as a threat. Other times the sandal is being wielded in the hand of a punter against a *hetaira*. Elsewhere we find them being beaten with sticks.

It is true that corporal punishment was more acceptable in ancient Greece than today. You will, for example, see on images of competing wrestlers the judge or judges standing by with whips or sticks clasped in their hands. You could argue there is a point here, that the use of physical punishment is designed to improve the athlete's performance, although Philostratus recounts several tales of athletes being killed by their trainers for underperforming, which it is less easy to get behind. The Spartan education system incorporated corporal punishment as an aid to producing an army composed of strong, fearless men. But where's the correction in these scenes of *hetairae* being beaten? The juxtaposition of sex and violence in these images is an uncomfortable one.

The life of a *hetaira* was not the comfortable, successful life some of our sources would have us believe. At the higher end of prostitution, they may have been but that still placed them towards the bottom of ancient Greek society, outsiders who would never gain admittance. Nowhere is this more clearly shown than in the life of Neaera.

A prostitute's story

I've repeatedly banged on about the bias in our sources towards the stories of men and the invisibility of women in ancient Greece; however, we do have an unusually full account of a Greek woman's life; her name was Neaera and in fifth-century BCE Athens she found herself entangled in a legal case.

The charge against Neaera was that of unlawful marriage, the law stated that only Athenian citizens could marry other Athenian citizens. Neaera's husband, Stephanus, was a citizen of Athens and Neaera also claimed this status. It was the prosecution's contention that Neaera was lying, she was no citizen of Athens, she couldn't be when her past life had been one of a prostitute. To prove their charge, the prosecution give one of the fullest accounts of a Greek woman's life available to us, and it is very telling on both how prostitution worked in antiquity and opens up a tantalising window into the thoughts, beliefs and prejudices that lurked in Greek women's minds.

One of the key themes the prosecution tackles is how the female citizenship will be tarnished by Neaera being included within its ranks. It's a theme which the prosecutor, Apollodorus, returns to with rhetorical flourish again and again.

> 'Well, what did you do?' And you will say, 'We acquitted her.' At this point the most virtuous of the women will be angry at you for having deemed it right that this woman should share in like manner with themselves in the public ceremonials and religious rites.[18]

In much the same way modern politicians like to bring their wives and daughters into political debates on women's issues as somehow proof that they are qualified to talk on the subject, Apollodorus appeals to the jurors, 'I would, then, have each one of you consider that he is casting his vote, one in the interest of his wife, one of his daughter, one of his mother, and one in the interest of the state and the laws and of religion, in order that these women may not be shown to be held in like esteem with the harlot.'[19]

Prostitutes, by virtue of their work, could never be respected or respectable citizens. To include them on the citizens' roll was to demean, according to Apollodorus, everything that a citizen of Athens was. There's a nastiness not so much lurking here as fully exposed in this line here from the same trial. 'And so they kept her and made use of her for as long as it pleased them. When they decided to marry however they informed her that they wished to see her, she who had been their personal sex companion.'[20]

Brothels may have been legal in Athens, young men may have been encouraged to visit them to release the overwhelming desires of youth, but the women who worked there were given very little consideration. They were playthings for men, men who were citizens and whose sexual acts did not damn them as they did the woman to a lifetime of being lesser. There's a whole series of these men who gleefully give evidence against Neaera recounting their activities with her in her prostitute days. There is no condemnation of them, no suggestion that their actions tarnish their citizen status, double standards loom so large as to keep us all in permanent shadow.

Prostitutes were therefore non-citizens, slaves and ex-slaves, foreigners and those born into the job or picked up after being abandoned by their parents by a brothel owner with vacancies to fill. Neaera's own background is grim, she was sold into her trade as a child.

> There were these seven girls who were purchased while they were small children by Nicarete, who was the freedwoman of Charisius the Elean and the wife of his cook Hippias. She was skilled in recognizing the budding beauty of young girls and knew well how to bring them up and train them artfully; for she made this her profession, and she got her livelihood from the girls.[21]

In the Corinthian brothel of Nicarete, Neaera attracts the attention of Timanoridas and Eucrates, who decide, given the amounts of money they were spending in Nicarete's brothel, that it would be cheaper in the long run to put their money together and buy Neaera outright. This is presented by Apollodorus as purely a financial decision, nowhere are any affections towards Neaera mentioned or any desire to save her from the life she was living.

They make use of Neaera until, as I mentioned in a quote a few lines previously, they decide to marry and Neaera needs to disappear. They pay her off, sort of. 'They offered, therefore, to remit one thousand drachmae toward the price of her freedom, five hundred drachmae apiece; and they bade her, when she found the means, to pay them the twenty minae.'[22] Twenty minae, for the record, is very roughly equivalent to 2,000 drachmae. So essentially these gentlemen agree to drop the price of what they think they would receive should they sell Neaera to another man or men and then demand 2,000 drachmae off her, which they hang about and wait for. What noble gentlemen!

Neaera finds the 2,000 drachmae by appealing to her patrons and to one Phrynion, who she begs for the final coins to make the full amount Eucrates and Timanoridas are demanding for her freedom. Of course, this now binds her to Phrynion who brings Neaera to Athens where life is still predictably grim for her, even though it might seem outwardly glamourous. Phrynion takes Neaera to parties where 'he had intercourse with her openly whenever and wherever he wished, making his privilege a display to onlookers'.[23]

The party of a celebrated charioteer newly returned from victory at the Pythian Games might sound like a glamorous event but here Neaera is dreadfully abused 'and in that place many had intercourse with her when she was drunk, while Phrynion was asleep, among them even the serving-men of Chabrias'.[24]

Did Phrynion, her companion, the man who took her to so many parties, defend her from these men or seek some sort of vengeance on her behalf for the rapes she suffered? No, he treated her with such 'wanton outrage' that Neaera packed up her stuff and left him.

It doesn't get much better for Neaera, I'm afraid, running away to Megara she runs into Stephanus and tells him her woeful story. Stephanus encourages Neaera to return to Athens with him, never mind about Phrynion, he tells her, full of bravado about what he would do to her former patron should he ever stumble across him. But Stephanus is no knight in shining armour. 'There were two reasons why he brought her here: first, because he would have a beautiful mistress without cost, and secondly, because her earnings would procure supplies and maintain the house; for he had no other income.'[25] What a gent!

Of course Phrynion reappears as a threat to Stephanus and Neaera's pose of being a couple of happily married Athenian citizens because he knows otherwise. He still owns Neaera, but he's quite happy to cut a deal with Stephanus.

> The terms were: that the woman should be free and her own mistress, but that she should give back to Phrynion all that she had taken with her from his house except the clothing and the jewels and the maid-servants; for these had been bought for the use of the woman herself; and that she should live with each of the men on alternate days.[27]

So Neaera is her own mistress and free, except for the clause whereby she is forced to share her body with two men. It's Timanoridas and Eucrates all over again, except that Neaera's declared free status means she doesn't benefit financially from this arrangement.

Neaera's story is fascinating on so many levels, it gives a real insight into how important class and citizenship was in ancient Athens. That Neaera has partaken in public rites and sacrifices to the gods that her real status barred her from goes beyond mere snobbery, it crosses into impiety and offences of the highest order.

Neaera's tale illustrates that prostitutes did not fit into one sole category and stay there. Neaera at times appears to have *hetairae* status, at other times she is much further down the ladder. Even when she appears to be at the high-class end of prostitution she is abused, taken to *symposia* as a live sex act and then raped by the guests. Her tale shows how utterly dependent she is on men, not just to pay for her services but to support her longer term, but such is her status that no man is going to stick by her, as is proven as she gets passed from patron to patron.

Neaera's tale is the negative of that of Aspasia, both are courted by powerful men but from one the powerful want advice, from the other they want control over her and sex. Both, however, share that outsider status.

The prosecution in the case against Neaera and Stephanus neatly sums up the rules for the different categories of women we have looked at in this section of the book.

> For this is what living with a woman as one's wife means – to have children by her and to introduce the sons to the members of the clan and of the deme, and to betroth the daughters to husbands as one's own. Mistresses we keep for the sake of pleasure, concubines for the daily care of our persons, but wives to bear us legitimate children and to be faithful guardians of our households.[28]

Part IV

Love is a Complicated Thing

Chapter 17

And Finally, to Love

How better to end this stroll through sex and sexuality in ancient Greece than with a subject that hasn't featured that often so far, love.

The goddess of love

In the first century CE, the endlessly curious Roman, Pliny the Elder, sat down to write his account of the world and everything in it. Pliny's *Natural Histories* is a stupendous work of literature which I beg all of you to read, because it is quite, quite brilliant. The *Natural Histories* is chock full of useful information from how to survive a shark attack: 'The only safe course is to turn on the sharks and frighten them. For sharks fear men just as much as men fear them.'[1] To selecting a wine: 'Wine from Pompeii are at their best within ten years and gain nothing from greater maturity.'[2] And on the far-away nation of China, which was 'well known for a woollen substance obtained from their forests',[3] which is most likely cotton.

Pliny has his fair share to say on art too. 'Superior to any other statue, not only to others made by Praxiteles himself, but throughout the world, is the Venus which many people sailed to Knidus to see.'[4] The Aphrodite of Knidus to which Pliny refers was the first depiction of the goddess Aphrodite in the nude, prior to this statue only male heroes and gods had been depicted nude, goddesses were always clothed. Praxiteles' innovation of a statue caused a sensation in the ancient world.

'Paris, Adonis, and Anchises saw me naked, Those are all I know of, but how did Praxiteles contrive it?'[5] wrote one poet at the time. Praxiteles' *Aphrodite* was a huge tourist attraction, so much so that when King Nicomedes of Bithynia offered to pay off Knidus' national debts if they would hand over their *Aphrodite* to him, the people of Knidus politely shook their head as one and kept taking those tourist drachmas, just as they had done for the five centuries before Pliny was gushing over their prize tourist attraction.

Pliny's account of the beauty of the *Aphrodite* statue is completely ruined and overshadowed by his inability to resist repeating this tale: 'There is a story that a man who had fallen in love with the statue hid in the temple at night and embraced it intimately, a stain bears witness to his lust.'[6] Ewww.

Praxiteles' original *Aphrodite* has been lost but luckily the Romans made numerous copies of her, so you too may see what so turned on Pliny's temple creeper in the Borghese Gallery in Florence, the Louvre in Paris, the British Museum in London or the Capitoline Museum in Rome, to name but a few of the museums who have a copy on display.

Praxiteles' innovation in art was taken up by others and two of the most famous works of art of all time feature the naked goddess. Leonardo di Vinci's *Mona Lisa* may attract the biggest crowds in the Louvre Museum but once they've ticked off that mysterious lady, they decamp to gather around another, the statue known as the *Venus de Milo*. Meanwhile, in the Uffizi Gallery in Florence, Italy tourists stand before and marvel at Botticelli's depiction of that goddess's birth and then rush down to buy their own version as depicted on postcards, tea towels, t-shirts, fridge magnets, pencil sharpeners and erasers in the gift shop.

In any European museum that has in its collection any ancient Greek or Italian art you will find an image of Aphrodite/Venus. A quick search on the British Museum website reveals 2,519 artefacts from the Classical era featuring Aphrodite/Venus, of which only 208 are on actual display. Included amongst those 208 items is a stunningly beautiful statue of the goddess crouching at her bath and another which has the perkiest set of buttocks I have ever seen – and I've looked at a great many museum bums. Aphrodite's buttocks are to be seen right across the world.

The beauty of Aphrodite as depicted by Praxiteles, Botticelli and many others distracts us from the goddess herself, we are consumed by the image rather than the person, or goddess in this case. Aphrodite may have been beautiful but like all Greek gods and goddesses she was involved in some ugly and unlovely acts in the name of love.

Even her birth, depicted so gloriously and cleanly by Botticelli, glosses over and beautifies the less than beautiful. Aphrodite was born from the sea as depicted by Botticelli, but more particularly she was born from white foam that had formed in the water after Kronos had thrown the castrated genitals of his father, Uranus, into the sea. Yep, you read that right, castrated genitals.

It's a story that the poet Hesiod references in his poem on the beginnings of the world, *The Theogony*. Male readers, you might want to cross your legs and initiate your best wincing face now. 'Himself from where he had been well concealed, stretched out one hand and with the other gripped the great, big, jagged sickle and then ripped his father's genitals off immediately and cast them down.'[7]

You are probably wondering what Uranus had done to deserve the loss of his man bits, and how the sea foam bit worked, and why you haven't heard this story before. I can supply you with the answers: (1) Because Uranus had developed a great hatred of all his children, and they feared for their lives. (2) Hesiod is rather vague about this, saying only 'they were swept away over the main a long time; and a white foam spread around them from the immortal flesh and in there grew a maiden',[8] which isn't terribly informative, and (3) because you likely learnt your Greek myths from a colourfully illustrated children's book from which this type of unlovely story tends not to feature.

Aphrodite was born from a dark act of would-be patricide and this darkness is recurrent in the myths in which she features. There were the women of Lemnos, whom she punished for not worshipping her with sufficient deference by making them smell so badly their husbands abandoned them for slave girls, the ultimate humiliation for a good Greek wife. The women took their revenge by killing every single one of their husbands except one, who must have been a busy chap for they had formed their own civilisation by the time Jason and his Argonaut crew stumbled upon them during their golden fleece quest.

Elsewhere we find Aphrodite's anger raised by Cenchreis, the Queen of Cyprus, who claimed her daughter, Myrrha, was more beautiful than the goddess. Aphrodite's wrath saw her curse Myrrha to fall in love with her own father, Cenchreis' husband King Cinyras. Myrrha's love for her father was so all-encompassing that she contrived to consummate her passion. She tricked Cinyras into sex by visiting him at night, and in the darkness giving herself to him repeatedly. There isn't much in the way of trickery required because Cinyras is apparently perfectly willing to sleep with anyone who should happen to turn up in his bedchamber with minimal questioning.

Myrrha fell pregnant with her father's child, which was when Cinyras discovered the identity of his secret midnight lover. Horrified by having had incestuous relations, he chased his daughter armed with a sword, and a terrified Myrrha begged the gods for assistance. The gods heard her plea and turned her into a myrrh tree, her tears forming the tree sap.

That's one hell of a revenge for one poorly considered but flippant comment. However, Aphrodite wasn't quite done yet messing with the Queen of Cyprus yet, as the ultimate 'screw you' the goddess later went on to have an affair with the offspring of this incest between Myrrha and Cinyras, the handsome Adonis. Which leaves us with a lot of questions, such as how did the now tree-Myrrha give birth? Why was Cinyras so amenable to an unknown woman breaking into his bedroom at night and demanding sex? And a more general 'What the hell?' at another tale left out of your illustrated Greek myths for children book.

In our society, love and falling in love is the subject of many a romcom film, romantic novel and newspaper article. Finding love is the goal for all in our society. We venerate and commemorate love on 14 February, St Valentine's Day. Ancient Greeks also commemorated love in festivals devoted to Aphrodite and her sons. But love to the ancient Greeks was not necessarily a good thing, there was a darkness at the heart of love. A love as dark as the birth of the goddess who personified it, lopped-off genitals and all.

Love, actually – is dark

That love was not necessarily a good thing is something Queen Helen of Sparta could well attest to. Incredibly beautiful, she had been married off to Menelaus, the King of Sparta, until in walked the Trojan prince, Paris. The intense rapture that followed saw her leave for Troy with Paris, something her husband, Menelaus, was distinctly unhappy about. So unhappy was Menelaus that he determined to get his wife back whatever the consequences, even if those consequences were a brutal ten-year war which diminished everyone morally and reputationally and led to the deaths of some top-drawer Greek heroes like Achilles and Hector.

Helen of Sparta was famously have said to have a face that had launched a thousand ships, it was probably far fewer that took her back to Sparta with her husband from Troy. Years later, she tells fellow Trojan War survivor, Odysseus, 'I sighed at the blindness Aphrodite had dealt me, drawing me there from my own dear country, abandoning daughter and bridal chamber, and a husband lacking neither in wisdom nor looks.'[9] Love had led Helen to abandon her duties, her very womanhood and had led to the collective madness of the war.

A poem from Greece's Archaic period (roughly 781–489 BCE) describes Aphrodite as 'a weaver of deceptions' who overwhelmed the 'high mindedness of mankind and there is no one in existence who is strong or wise enough to elude you'.[10] Socrates, as quoted in Xenophon's work *Symposium*, states that there were two Aphrodites, 'heavenly and vulgar'.[11] The vulgar Aphrodite excelled in looseness, the heavenly in chastity. 'One might conjecture, also, that different types of love come from different sources, carnal love from the "Vulgar" Aphrodite and from the "Heavenly" spiritual love, love of friendship and of noble conduct.'[12]

Aphrodite herself was a victim of love. Despite being married to the god Hephaestus, she embarked on an affair with the god of war, Ares. This was a liaison that ended in humiliation when the cuckolded husband contrived to trap the two lovers together under a net of gold and then invited all the other gods in to have a good laugh at them. You know love is a complicated thing when even the goddess that personifies it suffers its ill effects too.

The dark side of love

The love that Aphrodite inspired often led to dire consequences, but it is with her son, Eros, the product of that adulterous liaison with the god of war, that we see the madness of love most clearly. Eros has been sanitised for our culture, to us he's a podgy adorable cupid with a mop of blond curls and his bow and arrows ready to fire up love in an unsuspecting couple. The result is uniformly positive; the couple walk off hand in hand and live happily ever after. In Greek culture, Eros's arrows of love did not always produce this happy ending.

In Hesiod's tale of the formation of the world and all that dwell on her, Eros, the god of love, was born after chaos but before there was night or day, or all those long-limbed nymphs who populate Greek mythology. 'Eros fairest among the deathless gods, who unnerves the limbs and the wise counsels of all gods and all men within them.'[13] I am reminded of the regretful Helen of Sparta who lost her mind to love and the horrible consequences of that love madness that followed.

Other figures in mythology suffer from Eros' madness too. There was the hapless shepherd Hymnus, who, hit by Eros' arrow, fell deeply in love with the nymph Nicaea. The problem was that Nicaea did not love him back. The despondent and desperate Hymnus begged Nicaea to free him from the torment of his unrequited love for her by killing him. We must assume here that Hymnus had made an unbearable pest of himself to Nicaea, because she very readily takes him up on his offer and releases him bloodily from his torment.

This act of murdering her probable stalker angered Eros, who took his revenge on Nicaea by firing off another of his love arrows, this time into the god Dionysius. Dionysius was not the sad sack of a creature Hymnus had been and when he found himself rejected by Nicaea he certainly did not beg her to put him out of his misery. No, he drugged her and raped her instead. Remember this tale the next time you see Eros/Cupid as a cute podgy baby adorning Valentine's Day cards; he has a high body count.

Like Hymnus, the poet Anacreon similarly found the effects of Eros unpleasant. 'Again, Eros struck me like a blacksmith wielding an enormous hammer and bathed me in an ice-cold torrent.'[14] Spoke no one in a modern romcom ever. As academic James Davidson puts it in his book on Greeks and Greek love, 'One key aspect of Eros, however, is that he possesses the person in love. He is the daemon that puts your life off track, robs you of all your common sense and of sleep at night. He is very much an interior force, super-subjective, something you nurse inside you, getting your blood up, pushing and pestering, goading you with his whip driving you mad.'[15] Yikes.

Eros had several brothers, how many exactly changes from myth to myth, who served as gods of love with him. Pothos' particular realm of love was that of longing. Often the word *pothos* was used for non-romantic longing, such as the longing of the goddess Demeter for her daughter, Persephone, who had been abducted by the god of the underworld, Hades. Or Alexander the Great's longing to conquer new worlds. Socrates, as quoted by his fanboy Plato, sums this up: 'the word *pothos* signifies that it pertains not to that which is present, but to that which is elsewhere or absent'.[16]

With Alexander and Demeter, this was a non-romantic longing for that which is absent, but it could also be applied romantically. Post-Minotaur killing, the triumphant Theseus added in an island break at Naxos on route back home to Athens, presumably so everyone could use the toilet, stretch their legs a bit and so he could dump Ariadne, the woman who'd fallen in love with him and saved him from certain death in the labyrinth at the hands of a half-bull/half-man monster, and then sail off without her.

Theseus' heartless and ungrateful abandonment of Ariadne played out well for at least one person, or rather one god, Dionysius. We met him earlier in this book driving women into murderous mobs; he did not do so with Ariadne, which I for one am glad of. Discovering her alone on the island and suffering greatly with *pothos*, that dreadful longing form of love for someone you can't have (because he's a shit of man who's sailed off with his mates because you're cramping his style), the smooth Dionysius enters with one hell of a chat-up line. 'Maiden, why do you sorrow for the deceitful man of Athens? Let pass the memory of Theseus; you have Dionysos for your lover, a husband incorruptible for the husband of a day! If you are pleased with the mortal body of a youthful years mate, Theseus can never challenge Dionysos in manhood or comeliness.'[17] Good line it may have been but Dionysius still required the services of Eros to pincushion Ariadne with arrows to make her susceptible to his 'hey, I'm a god, you'll never do any better than me' patter.

Another brother to Eros was Himeros. Himeros was the god of sexual desire, of captivation and also of getting it on. *Pothos* was what Ariadne was drenched in after Theseus had buggered off and left her, Himeros was who popped up when Dionysius discovered her on her island. Longing for what was absent, followed by meeting and falling for someone new. There are several vases that depict the god Himeros floating about Dionysius and Ariadne, ready to offer his assistance in helping them to get it on.

But like Eros and Pothos before him, Himeros' powers were not necessarily a good thing nor a welcome thing. You could be the unwanted subject of sexual desire or suffer from sexual desire for someone who did not want you. Mythology is awash with tales, such as Daphne, who was relentlessly pursued by the god Apollo and, like Myrra before, was transformed into a tree by the gods to escape her pursuer. Although this didn't work out so well for Daphne, as Apollo, finding his beloved was now a laurel tree, adopted the laurel tree as his sacred plant, so she was never truly free of him.

One version of this tale has Apollo's aggressive love for Daphne being the result of one of Eros' arrows, a revenge for Apollo's mocking of the love god's skill as an archer. From which we might again note that mocking or insulting the gods is a very bad move, even if you are a god yourself.

Eros, Pothos and Himeros together are the Erotes, the winged gods of love. Occasionally these three have companions such as Anteros who symbolises mutual love and Hedylogus, the god of sweet-talking and flattery, as light to their potential darkness. Although even mutual love, when you think about it, can have a dark side, a love that can inspire horrific acts and sweet-talk and flattery is the bane of many a woman's life who just wants to get on with her weekly supermarket shop without being harassed. The Greeks were onto something here, there is no form of love that doesn't have a dark side.

Gaining love by any means necessary

The gods didn't have a monopoly on inspiring love where no love had previously been, the individual citizen could take matters into their own hands and acquire love for themselves. If you're thinking of flowers and chocolates, sweet notes and a general positioning of yourself as a good prospect for fumbling about with, I'm afraid I am about to disappoint you once again. Nor am I talking about nipping down the temple with something special for Eros and Aphrodite like a votive offering of some nice pottery or an enormous white bull with the hope that they will feel well-disposed enough towards you that you'll get a bit of a snog out of it from that girl you fancy. No, the ancient Greeks had something far more practical than appealing to the gods or nice gestures to bring a bit of love into your life; they had magic.

Magic to us in the twenty-first century is men in frilly shirts pulling doves out of their sleeves or accosting people quietly minding their own business walking down the street and forcing them to participate in card tricks; it's a form of entertainment. In antiquity, magic was much more practical and useful. I personally have never found myself in a situation where it has been necessary for me to produce a rabbit from out of a top hat, I'm 50 so I'm not completely ruling it out yet but so far it's just not cropped up. Greek magic, on the other hand, is far more applicable to the every day, we've all had a headache that wouldn't shift, a relative with a short fuse, wanted to know if we or a loved one is up the duff or simply wanted to inflict an 'evil sleep' on someone (who hasn't?). These are all things that magic could take care of as well as love.

Love is a universally felt emotion, so it is unsurprising that it features so heavily in spells and magic. The *Magical Papyri* collection of spells has nineteen 'love spells for attraction' and twenty-seven general 'love spells' listed alongside instructions on how to make love charms and love potions. Love was big business in the magical world

Love spells tend to involve gathering some specified items together and then chanting a prescribed set of words. Some love spells, it has to be said, rated as easy on the magical scale, a first-year homework assignment that even Ron Weasley could complete without begging help off Hermione, for example: 'For love say while kissing passionately: "I – am THAZI N EPIBATHA CHEOUCH CHA I am I am CHARIEMOUTH LAILAM."'[18] Although admittedly this spell is dependent on you having pulled the object of your affection already, which Ron Weasley might struggle with, and sealing the deal on a lifetime of kissing passionately.

Other spells you are going to struggle to emulate in the twenty-first century, such as this one that requires you to

> leave a little of the bread which you eat; break it up and form it into seven bite-size pieces. And go to where heroes and gladiators and those who have died a violent death were slain. / Say the spell to the pieces of bread and throw them. And pick up some polluted dirt from the place where you perform the ritual and throw it inside the house of the woman whom you desire, go on home and go to sleep.[19]

I mean you could try going to the modern equivalent of an amphitheatre, a football stadium with your pieces of bread but even if you say all 653 words on the prescribed incantation perfectly, given that very few football matches end with anyone being violently slain your love spell isn't going to work.

Other love spells involve ingredients you might just struggle to find in your local high street. The bread from the above spell is no problem to source, cumin is on the shelf of any supermarket (although you might have to live in the trendier part of town to get specifically Ethiopian cumin), milk, again, no problem, and even frankincense and myrrh you could likely find courtesy of some posh soap shop or perfumery. Things that love spells require that you might struggle to find include a virgin goat (food labelling in the UK does not yet specify the sexual history of your cut of meat); the skin of an ass is a very specialised request for your local butcher that is going to raise his eyebrows even higher than that time you asked him whether he thought the goat was popular with, like, lady goats and you are not going to be finding any spotted lizards anytime soon in the British countryside.

Sourcing ingredients is not the only difficulty, the incantations that go with the ingredients are long, very long and sometimes require you to sit in a bath whilst saying them, or throw apples up in the air whilst chanting or be up at the third hour of the night specifically when you'd much rather be in bed. I have a sense that spells are so complicated and difficult to meet buyer expectations, you'd want to know you were getting your money's worth of magic. The more elaborate the spell, the more potent it likely felt to the buyer. Certainly spells for curing a headache are a lot less complicated than the love spells in the *Magical Papyri*, even a migraine headache can be cured by this simple spell. 'Take oil in your hands and utter the spell: "Zeus sowed grape seed: it parts the soil; he does not sow it; it does not sprout."'[20] Though please don't throw away your painkillers yet.

Not only are the incantations used in love spells long, they can also be downright disturbing.

> Go stand above her (NN) head and take Away from her sweet sleep. And never let Eyelid come glued to eyelid, but let her Be sore distressed with wakeful cares for me. And if she lies with someone else in her Embrace, let her thrust him away and take Me in her heart. Let her abandon him At once and stand before my door subdued In soul at longing for my bed of love.[21]

This does not sound like a healthy love being expressed here, the spell maker wants the object of his affection to suffer before she is drawn to him.

Here's another spell that asks the same, that the beloved must suffer and the spell maker be the only source of relief:

> Myrrh, and go into every place and seek out her, NN, and open her right side and enter like thunder, like lightning, like a burning flame, and make her thin, [pale,] weak, limp, incapable of [action] in [any part of her body] until she leaps forth and comes to me, NN, son of NN (add the usual, whatever you wish). Immediately, immediately; quickly, quickly.[22]

You can feel the desperation in the words, but then people resorting to magic to acquire love are likely to be desperate, perhaps this is their last chance as they see it after every normal attempt to gain their affection has failed. The phrases used in incantations certainly speak to the desperate and scorned who essentially want control over someone else, for this is, when we boil it down, what a love spell is intended to do. A love spell is intended to control and induce feelings in another person, it is that dark side to love that we explored earlier in the chapter.

Aside from love spells, there are a number of spells that talk of binding someone to you, now these get very dark. 'Do this, bind her for all the time of my life and help force her, NN to be serviceable to me, NN, and let her not frolic away from me for even one hour of life.'[23] This is no healthy love, this is the love that a stalker has for his prey, possessive and cruel. This same spell also involves making a clay model of his love and then the instructions are to

> take thirteen copper needles and stick 1 in the brain while saying, 'I am piercing your brain, NN'; and stick 2 in the ears and 2 in the eyes and 1 in the mouth and 2 in the midriff and 1 in the hands and 2 in the pudenda and 2 in the soles, saying each time, 'I am piercing such and such a member of her, NN, so that she may remember no one but me, NN, alone.'[24]

This is not nice stuff.

There were evidently laws against the use of magic to harm others, although the spells I've mentioned so far evidently did not qualify as harm, controlling in a very disturbing way, yes, but physical harm, no. There is mention in a trial speech of Demosthenes of the execution of someone using magic: 'It was this brother – I pass over the other facts – who got possession of the drugs and charms from the servant of Theoris of Lemnos, the filthy sorceress whom you put to death on that account with all her family.'[25]

Talking of love

Having gone over to the dark side, let us leap back into the light and talk about the positives of love. Or rather we shall let those guests at Plato's *symposium* sum it up for us in one final rhetorical flourish, over to you, boys.

> Phaedrus: 'Love is the most ancient and revered of the gods, and supreme when it comes to the human acquisition of excellence and blessedness in life and after death.'[26]
>
> Pausanias: 'This is the Love belonging to the Heavenly goddess. It too is heavenly and of great value to the city and the citizenry, compelling the lover himself, and the beloved, to pay much attention to excellence.'[27]
>
> Aristophanes: 'Each of us is a counterpart of a human being, since we have been cut in half and are like flat-fish, two produced from one, each constantly searching for the particular counterpart of itself.'[28]
>
> Socrates: 'Whoever is touched by Love becomes a poet even if he had previously been devoid of the Muse.'[29]

Or perhaps the writer of a book on sex and sexuality in your day, Socrates.

Author's Note

Like its predecessor, *Sex and Sexuality in Ancient Rome*, this is not an academic work, nor is it an in-depth examination of the topic. Rather this book is written for every person out there who always fancied knowing a bit more about sex in ancient Greece but didn't know where to start. It is an introduction to some of the themes around sex and sexuality in ancient Greece rather than a comprehensive account of every aspect of the topic.

My intention whilst writing both books is that they serve as a springboard that launches the reader off into their own further study. Or alternatively to slam shut the cover and put the book face down on their coffee table, having decided they now know more than they ever wish to about sex and sexuality in ancient times. It can go either way.

For those of you who stuck with it to the end, I thank you.

L. J. Trafford, May 2025

Notes

Part I: Understanding Ancient Greece

Introduction: Greeks Bearing Gifts

1. *Sex and Sexuality in Ancient Rome* by L. J. Trafford is also available from Pen and Sword Books. It is a cracking read.
2. Hippocrates was a doctor from the island of Kos who is credited with being the first physician in history who was actually any good at curing people. Though he did not contribute anything to the collection of medical texts known as the Hippocratic Corpus, his influence can be felt oozing out of the pages written by his acolytes. Of works actually written by Hippocrates himself we have none. Although if you visit the island of Kos you will find a tree there that the locals claim Hippocrates sat under to think deeply serious thoughts and write all those books that we do not have. Except he probably didn't because the tree isn't nearly as old as it needs to be to be contemporary with Hippocrates.
3. The most controversial of these being the friezes that were chipped off the Parthenon and sold to a certain Lord Elgin. This collection of statues, known as the Elgin Marbles, is currently housed in the British Museum in London and remains the subject an ongoing dispute between the British and Greek governments. See this article from BBC News to get the current position (as of 4 December 2024) on the marbles: www.bbc.co.uk/news/entertainment-arts-30342462
4. Percy Bysshe Shelley, *Hellas*, Preface.
5. Lord George Gordon Byron, *Byron Childe Harold's Pilgrimage*, Canto the Second II.1.
6. James Stewart and Nicholas Revette, *The Art and Architecture of Ancient Greece*, introduction.
7. In the 1870s German businessman and self-promoter Henrich Schliemann claimed to have discovered Troy near the town of Hissarlik in Turkey. He'd discovered something certainly, but in his haste and excitement it likely wasn't the Troy of the Trojan War because he'd bulldozed straight through that layer of archaeological finds. Schliemann was not your white-gloved, delicate brush type of archaeologist.
8. Aristophanes, *Thesmophoriazusae*, 252, George Theodoridis' 2007 translation.
9. As featured in Shakespeare's *The Winter's Tale*.
10. Chapter 1. The Basics.
11. Herodotus, *Histories*, VIII.144.2.
12. See this article: www.rom.on.ca/en/blog/the-evans-connection-part-2-the-minoans-created
13. Periods of Greek pottery include the geometric which were fashionable around 1000–700 BCE, the orientalising period when Greek potters were influenced by goods coming their direction from the Near East between 700 and 600 BCE and the later Archaic and Classical periods which get subdivided into black figure, red figure and white ground based on the types of pottery discovered.

Part II: Men

Chapter 2: The Body Beautiful

1. Philostratus, *Gymnasticus*, 25.
2. Aristophanes, *The Clouds*, 1007.
3. Aristophanes, *The Clouds*.
4. Thucydides, *The History of the Peloponnesian War*, V 1.6.5.
5. Plato, *The Republic*, Book V, 452x.
6. Xenophon, *Hellenica*, Book III 4.19.
7. Pliny the Elder, *The Natural Histories*, XV.19.
8. Plato, *Laws*, VII.1.
9. Ibid.
10. Plato, *Laws*, VII.
11. Philostratus, *Gymnasticus*, 19.
12. Xenophon, *Memorabilia*, Book III.12.1.
13. Xenophon, *Memorabilia*, Book III.12.5.
14. Xenophon, *Memorabilia*, Book III.12.6.
15. Xenophon, *Memorabilia*, Book III.12.5.
16. Chapter 3. The Ultimate Perfection: Athletes.
17. Philostratus, *Gymnasticus*, 1.
18. Ibid.
19. Philostratus, *Gymnasticus*, 2.
20. Philostratus, *Gymnasticus*, 14.
21. Philostratus, *Gymnasticus*, 25.
22. Philostratus, *Gymnasticus*, 28.
23. Philostratus, *Gymnasticus*, 56.
24. Philostratus, *Gymnasticus*, 14.
25. Philostratus, *Gymnasticus*, 21.
26. Philostratus, *Gymnasticus*, 18.
27. Philostratus, *Gymnasticus*, 18.
28. Philostratus, *Gymnasticus*, 18.
29. Suetonius, *Life of Nero*, 22.
30. Michael B. Poliakoff, *Combat Sports in the Ancient World*, p. 12.
31. Poliakoff, *Combat Sports in the Ancient World*, p. 19.
32. Philostratus, *Gymnasticus*, 1.
33. Pausanias, *Tour of Greece*, 6.18.
34. Pausanias, *Tour of Greece*, 6.3.15.
35. Pausanias, *Tour of Greece*, 6.4.3.
36. Pausanias, *Tour of Greece*, 6.5.1.
37. From the official Olympics website, www.olympics.com, where you will find a wealth of statistics that'll kill the hours you could have spent down the gym getting fit.
38. Pausanias, *Tour of Greece*, 6.14.6.
39. Pliny the Elder, *Natural Histories*, Book VII.83.
40. Morrocco made the final sixteen teams in 1986 and memorably came fourth in the 2022 tournament. Which is not a bad record given they have only played in six World Cups.
41. Philostratus, *Gymnasticus*, 24.

42. Pausanias, *Tour of Greece*, 8.40.3–4.
43. As quoted on https://olympians.org/woa/olympism
44. Plato, *Laws*, VII.
45. Xenophon, *Memorabilia*, Book III.12.5.
46. The Athenian citizens were divided into ten tribes. Each tribe was represented in the Assembly and could be called up en masse by tribe for any military threats.
47. Xenophon, *Cyropaedia*, Book 1.18.
48. The Parthenon is one of Greece's most recognisable historical buildings: a temple dedicated to the goddess Athena which also served as a treasury.
49. Philostratus, *Gymnasticus*, 1.

Chapter 4: Bodily Perfection the Spartan Way

1. After expelling the Persians from Greece, several of the islands were closer to the Persian Empire than they felt comfortable with and so an offer from the victorious Athenian navy to act as their protector was welcome. The Delian League, as this arrangement was known, was a mutually protective consortium of Greek city states who each paid a sort of membership fee. This membership fee soon became what was effectively tribute payable to Athens, or else. It was the 'or else' more than anything that pulled the rug from under the feet of the Delian League members who now found themselves part of an Athenian empire. It was an appeal from the members of this new empire to the Spartans to help free them from Athenian control that kicked off the Peloponnesian War.
2. Plutarch, *Sayings of the Spartans*.
3. Plutarch, *Sayings of the Spartans*.
4. https://uk.spartan.com/en/race/ultra
5. Paul Cartledge, *The Spartans*, p. 23.
6. Aelian, *Various Histories*, Book 14: Chapter 7.
7. Aelian, *Various Histories*, Book 14: Chapter 8.
8. Plutarch, *Life of Lycurgus*, 1.
9. Although he probably wasn't because Homer is more fictitious than Lycurgus is.
10. Soranus, *Gynaecology*, 2.10.79.
11. Plutarch, *Life of Lycurgus*, 16.1.
12. Plutarch, *Life of Lycurgus*, 16.1.
13. See this article by Bad Ancient: www.badancient.com/claims/spartans-throw-babies-mountains
14. The counterpoint to this is the case of the English king, Richard III. Fans of Richard have long argued that the representation of him by historians and Shakespeare as a murderous king deformed by a hunchback was Tudor propaganda to blacken his character. Astonishingly in 2012 the remains of Richard III were discovered beneath a carpark in the city of Leicester. The skeleton showed that Richard III suffered from scoliosis, which had caused his spine to curve, and so proved that those historians had been entirely correct in describing him as a having a hunchback and we should all have believed them in the first place.
15. Plutarch, *The Customs of the Spartans*, 19.
16. Xenophon, *Constitution of the Lacedaemonians*, 1.
17. Agesilaus ruled Sparta from 400–360 BCE during the Peloponnesian Wars in which Sparta was victorious.

18. Xenophon, *Constitution of the Lacedaemonians*, 2.
19. Xenophon, *Constitution of the Lacedaemonians*, 2.4.
20. Ibid.
21. Plutarch, *Life of Lycurgus*, 18.1.
22. How Sparta was able to maintain what was effectively a military state was because they had enslaved the entire population of Messina, which neighboured Sparta. The enslaved Messenians, known as Helots, acted as the farmers and food producers Sparta needed.
23. Myke Coles' book, *The Bronze Lie*, pulls apart the Spartan image.

Chapter 5: Greek Love

1. Plato, *Symposium*, 176.
2. Plato, *Symposium*, 177.
3. Plato, *Symposium*, 178d.
4. Plato, *Symposium*, 179b.
5. Plato, *Symposium*, 183e.
6. Plato, *Symposium*, 185b.
7. Plato, *Symposium*, 178e–179a.
8. Plato, Symposium, 181b.
9. E. M. Forster, *Maurice*, Chapter 9.
10. E. M. Forster, *Maurice*, Part 2, Chapter 12.
11. Sentencing Statement of Justice Wills: www.famous-trials.com/wilde/335-statement
12. Ibid.
13. Plato, *Symposium*, 178c.
14. Plato, *Symposium*, 191c.
15. Testimony by Oscar Wilde.
16. Aeschines, *Against Timarchus*, 1.135.
17. Plutarch, *Life of Alcibiades*, 1.3.
18. Plutarch, *Life of Alcibiades*, 4.
19. See www.worcester.ac.uk/about/news/academic-blog/health-and-wellbeing-blogs/the-importance-of-positive-male-role-models.aspx for just one example looking at the importance of role models for young men.
20. Plutarch, *Life of Alcibiades*, 4.
21. Plato, *Symposium*, 184e.
22. Plato, *Symposium*, 185.
23. Plato, *Phaedrus*, 232E.
24. Plato, *Phaedrus*, 233A.
25. As quoted in *Love, Sex and Marriage in Ancient Greece* by Nikolaos A. Vrisimtzis, who points out anal sex is depicted on vases in heterosexual couplings.
26. Plutarch, *Life of Alcibiades*, 4.
27. Aeschines, *Against Timarchus*, 1.21.
28. Aeschines, *Against Timarchus*, 1.155.
29. Aeschines, *Against Timarchus*, 1.93.
30. Aeschines, *Against Timarchus*, 1.55.
31. Aeschines, *Against Timarchus*, 1.30.
32. Plato, *Symposium*, 181d.
33. Nikolaos A. Vrisimtzis, *Love, Sex and Marriage in Ancient Greece*, introduction to Chapter 10.

34. From the NAMBLA website.
35. https://ianpace.wordpress.com/2014/02/26/pie-documentary-evidence-2-from-magpie-1-8-trigger-warning-contains-disturbing-material
36. Testimony of Charles Parker during Wilde's trial.
37. Aechines, *Against Timarchus*, 1.9.
38. Ibid.
39. Ibid.
40. Aechines, *Against Timarchus*, 1.3.
41. James Davidson, *The Greeks and Greek Love*, p. 81.
42. See https://research.reading.ac.uk/research-blog/2020/07/13/children-arent-starting-puberty-younger-medieval-skeletons-reveal as an example.
43. Plutarch, *Life of Solon*.

Chapter 6: Greek Love Outside of Athens

1. Xenophon, *Constitution of Lacedaemonians*, 2.14.
2. Xenophon, *Constitution of Lacedaemonians*, 2.14.
3. Xenophon, *Constitution of Lacedaemonians*, 2.14.
4. Cicero, *The Republic*, 3.3.
5. Xenophon, *Constitution of Lacedaemonians*, 2.14.
6. Xenophon, *Constitution of Lacedaemonians*, 6.1.
7. Xenophon, *Constitution of Lacedaemonians*, 6.2.
8. Xenophon, *Constitution of Lacedaemonians*, 2.2.
9. Xenophon, *Constitution of Lacedaemonians*, 2.10.
10. Plutarch, *Life of Lycurgus*, 15.3.
11. Plutarch, *Life of Lycurgus*, 15.3.
12. Cartledge, *The Spartans*, p. 158–159.
13. Strabo, *Geography*, Book X, Chapter 4, 15.
14. Strabo, *Geography*, Book X, Chapter 4.17.
15. Strabo, *Geography*, Book X, Chapter 4.21.
16. Strabo, *Geography*, Book X, Chapter 4.21.
17. Ibid.
18. Ibid.
19. Ibid.
20. Ibid.
21. Ibid.
22. Plato, *Laws*, Book 1.
23. Plato, *Symposium*, 182b.
24. Cicero, *The Republic*, 3.4.4.
25. Xenophon, *Hellenica*, 3.5.
26. Ibid.
27. Plutarch, *Life of Pelopidas*, 20.3.
28. Plutarch, *Life of Pelopidas*, 4.2.
29. Plato, *Symposium*, 173e.
30. Plutarch, *Life of Pelopidas*, 4.5.
31. Plutarch, *Life of Pelopidas*, 4.3.
32. Plutarch, *Life of Pelopidas*, 18.1.
33. Vrisimtzis, *Love, Sex and Marriage in Ancient Greece*, 1090.

34. Vrisimtzis, *Love, Sex and Marriage in Ancient Greece*, location 109.
35. Straton, 12.5.
36. Straton, 12.192.
37. Straton, 2.9.
38. Straton, 12.205.
39. Straton, 12.222.
40. Arrian, *History of Alexander*, Chapter XIV.
41. Arrian, *History of Alexander*, Chapter XIV.
42. Sexual Offences Act 2003, 21.2.

Chapter 7. Boys Will Be Boys – The Symposium

1. https://dictionary.cambridge.org/dictionary/english/symposium
2. For example, the Symposium held by the Bioelectric Department at Cambridge University, the titles of whose talks are beyond the comprehension of the layman, let alone the actual content of them. *3D printing PEDOT and eutectogels conductive polymers for bioelectronics, stimuli-responsive organic conductors and conductive polymer bioelectronics: Towards fully polymeric devices.* I am sure I speak for every non-expert when I say, sorry, you what?
3. Vrisimtzis, *Love, Sex and Marriage in Ancient Greece*, 1019.
4. Demosthenes, *Against Neaera*, 59.33.
5. Xenophon, *Symposium*, 14.
6. Xenophon, *Symposium*, 14.
7. Xenophon, *Symposium*, 7.
8. Xenophon, *Symposium*, 10.
9. Xenophon, *Symposium*, 12.

Chapter 8: Penises

1. https://web.stanford.edu/~eckert/PDF/PenisTesticlesSlang.pdf
2. Mark Haskell Smith, *Rude Talk in Athens*, p. 30.
3. Euripides, *The Bacchae*, 270.
4. Euripides, *The Bacchae*, 451.
5. Euripides, *The Bacchae*, 1120.
6. Pisistratus ruled as a tyrant of Athens during 546–527 BCE.
7. Aristophanes, *The Acharnians*, 241.
8. Aristophanes, *The Acharnians*, 241.
9. Aristophanes, *The Thesmophoriazusae*, 81.
10. Euripides, *Cyclops*, 165.
11. Euripides, *Cyclops*, 366.
12. Aristophanes, *Lysistrata*, 1.
13. Aristophanes, *The Knights*, 30.
14. Aristophanes, *The Assembly Women*, 1015.
15. Aristophanes, *Thesmophoriazusa*, 643.
16. Aristophanes, *Lysistrata*, 1143.
17. Plutarch, *Life of Alcibiades*, 17.3.
18. Ibid.
19. Plutarch, *Life of Alcibiades*, 18.
20. Thucydides, *History of the Peloponnesian War*, Book vi.27.

21. Thucydides, *History of the Peloponnesian War*, Book v.28.
22. Plutarch, *Life of Alcibiades*, 18.4.
23. Plutarch, *Life of Alcibiades*, 18.4.

Part III: Women

Chapter 9: A Punishment from the Gods

1. The Old Testament, Genesis, 27.
2. The Old Testament, Genesis, 31.
3. Quran, 15.29.
4. Hesiod, *Works and Days*, 43–54.
5. Hesiod, *Works and Days*, 59–60.
6. Hesiod, Works and Days, 64.
7. Hesiod, *Works and Days*, 65–66.
8. Hesiod, *Works and Days*, 66–68.
9. Hesiod, *Works and Days*, 91.
10. Hesiod, *Theogony*, 590–612.
11. Hesiod, *Works and Days*, 597.
12. Hesiod, *Works and Days*, 375.
13. https://en.wikipedia.org/wiki/Types_of_Women
14. Semonides, *Poem 7: Types of Women*, 1.
15. Semonides, *Poem 7: Types of Women*, 12.
16. Ibid.
17. Semonides, *Poem 7: Types of Women*, 43–44.
18. Semonides, *Poem 7: Types of Women*, 93.
19. Semonides, *Poem 7: Types of Women*, 72.
20. Archilochos, P.Colon, 7511.
21. Chapter 10. Wives – Sharing the Burden or the Cause of It?
22. Hesiod, *Works and Days*, 536–563.
23. Hesiod, *Works and Days*, 722–723.
24. Hesiod, *Works and Days*, 721.
25. Hesiod, *Works and Days*, 293–319.
26. Hesiod, *Works and Days*, 695–700.
27. Hesiod, *Works and Days*, 695–705.
28. Semonides, *Poem 7: Types of Women*, 26.
29. Xenophon, *Memorabilia*, 2.2.4.
30. Xenophon, *Economic*, 3.15.
31. Xenophon, *Economic*, 3.10.
32. Xenophon, *Economic*, 3.10.
33. Xenophon, *Symposium*, 11.
34. Xenophon, *Symposium*, 11.
35. Plutarch, *Advice to Bride and Groom*, introduction.
36. Plutarch, *Advice to Bride and Groom*, 3.
37. Plutarch, *Advice to Bride and Groom*, 4.
38. Plutarch, *Advice to Bride and Groom*, 4.
39. Plutarch, *Advice to Bride and Groom*, 13.
40. Plutarch, *Advice to Bride and Groom*, 15.

41. Plutarch, *Advice to Bride and Groom*, 5.
42. Plutarch, *Advice to Bride and Groom*, 16.
43. Plutarch, *Advice to Bride and Groom*, 30.
44. Xenophon, *Economics*, 2.10.
45. Aristotle, *Politics*, Book 7, 16.
46. Plutarch, *Life of Solon*, 20.4.
47. The exception being poor women who have always worked because of necessity.
48. Demosthenes, *Against Neaera*, 59.8.
49. James Robson, *Sex and Sexuality in Classical Athens*, p. 11.
50. Plutarch, *Life of Aristides*, 27.
51. Demosthenes, *Against Neaera*, 59.113.
52. Isaeus, *On the Estate of Pyrrhus*, 3.8.
53. Isaeus, *On the Estate of Pyrrhus*, 3.9.
54. Plutarch, *On the Bravery of Women*, 242 e11.
55. Aristophanes, *The Assembly Women*, 111.
56. Thucydides, *History of the Peloponnesian War*, Book 2 xix.2.
57. Sophocles, *Ajax*, 293.
58. Homer, *The Odyssey*.
59. Euripides, *The Trojan Women*, 654–5 5.4.
60. Plutarch, *Moralia*, 32.1.

Chapter 11: Women's Lives

1. Isacus, *On the Estate of Pyrrhus*, 3.13–4.
2. Euripides, *Medea*, 1.7–1.10.
3. Aristotle, *Economics*, 3.1.
4. Lysias, *Against Simon*, 3.3–7.
5. Xenophon, *Economics*, 9.5.
6. Plutarch, *Life of Solon*, 8.3.
7. Plutarch, *Life of Solon*, 10.
8. Plutarch, *Life of Solon*, 11.1.
9. Plutarch, *Life of Solon*, 13.1.
10. Plutarch, Life of Solon, 14.5.
11. Plutarch, *Life of Solon*, 21.
12. Plutarch, *Life of Solon*, 23.1.
13. Plato, *Laws*, Book VI.II.
14. Ibid.
15. Ibid.
16. Ibid.
17. Ibid.
18. Plato, *Laws*, Book VI.II.
19. Aristotle, *Politics*, 2.6.
20. Aristotle, *Politics*, 2.9.
21. Demosthenes, *Against Neaera*, 3.122.
22. P. Walcot, 'Greek Attitudes Towards Women: The Mythological Evidence', *Greece & Rome*, vol. 31, no. 1, 1984, pp. 37–47. *JSTOR*, www.jstor.org/stable/642368. Accessed 18 May 2025.

23. Shima Tabatabai and Nasser Simforoosh, *Health Care and Medical Education to Promote Women's Health in Iran: Four Decades Efforts, Challenges and Recommendations.*
24. Kamelia Aryafar, 'How Iranian immigrants can be role models for diversity in STEM', 5 February 2020, https://thehill.com/changing-america/opinion/481684-how-iranian-immigrants-can-be-role-models-for-diversity-in-stem
25. Lysias, *On the Murder of Eratosthenes*, 1.
26. Lysias, *On the Murder of Eratosthenes*, 8.
27. Lysias, *On the Murder of Eratosthenes*, 50.
28. Lysias, *On the Murder of Eratosthenes*, 1.
29. Lysias, *On the Murder of Eratosthenes*, 9.
30. Lysias, *On the Murder of Eratosthenes*, 9.
31. Lysias, *On the Murder of Eratosthenes*, 10.
32. Lysias, *On the Murder of Eratosthenes*, 12.
33. Lysias, *On the Murder of Eratosthenes*, 16.
34. Lysias, *On the Murder of Eratosthenes*, 24.
35. Lysias, *On the Murder of Eratosthenes*, 29.
36. Lysias, *On the Murder of Eratosthenes*, 27.
37. Lysias, *On the Murder of Eratosthenes*, 31.
38. See Sarah B. Pomeroy, *Goddesses, Whores, Wives and Slaves*, p. 86.
39. Pomeroy, *Goddesses, Whores, Wives and Slaves*, p. 86.
40. Demosthenes, *Against Eubulides*, 57.30.
41. Demosthenes, *Against Eubulides*, 57.34.
42. Demosthenes, *Against Eubulides*, 57.35.
43. Xenophon, *Memorabilia*, 2.7.
44. Xenophon, *Memorabilia*, 2.7.
45. Xenophon, *Memorabilia*, 2.7.

Chapter 12: Women Outside of Athens

1. Gortyn Code, IV.
2. Gortyn Code, XIV.
3. Ibid.
4. Gortyn Code, V.
5. Gortyn Code, X.
6. Xenophon, *Constitution of the Lacedaemonians*, 9.
7. Xenophon, *Constitution of the Lacedaemonians*, 5.
8. Xenophon, *Constitution of the Lacedaemonians*, 5.
9. Xenophon, *Constitution of the Lacedaemonians*, 4.
10. Xenophon, *Constitution of the Lacedaemonians*, 9.
11. Plutarch, *Sayings of Spartan Women*, Gorgo 5.
12. Plutarch, *Sayings of Spartan Women*, Other Spartan women of fame unknown 2.
13. Aristotle, *Politics*, 2.9.
14. Xenophon, *Constitution of the Lacedaemonians*, 3.
15. Xenophon, *Constitution of the Lacedaemonians*, 3.
16. Xenophon, *Constitution of the Lacedaemonians*, 5.7.
17. Marguerite Johnson, *Sexuality in Greek and Roman Society and Literature*, p. 113; Athenaeus, 602d.
18. Plutarch, *Life of Lycurgus*, 3.5.

Chapter 13: What Little Girls Are Made Of

1. According to the website of the Cleveland Clinic based in Cleveland, Ohio, USA: https://health.clevelandclinic.org/reiki
2. According to another wellness practitioner website: https://familytreeacuwell.com/acupuncture-centennial
3. Galen, *Mixtures*, 2.4.
4. Hippocrates, *Aphorisms*, Section V, part 57.
5. Aristotle, *On the Generation of Animals*, 76b 19–22.
6. Aristotle, *On the Generation of Animals*, 15/89.
7. Ibid.
8. Hippocrates, *On Diseases of Women*, 1.6, L. VIII.30.
9. Ibid.
10. Plato, *Timaeus*.
11. Ibid.
12. Ibid.
13. Pure speculation, it could be that puppies come in a litter and so were used to aid fertility or that dead meat of whatever source tends to be moist (and moistness, as we've seen, was a good thing).
14. Soranus, *Gynaecology*, 3.29.

Chapter 14: Men, Women and Sex

1. Hesiod, *Works and Days*, 810–813.
2. Plutarch, *Advice to Bride and Groom*, 2.1.
3. Plutarch, *Advice to Bride and Groom*, 7.1.
4. Ovid, *Metamorphoses*, Book 3.316.
5. Ovid, *Metamorphoses*, Book 3.316.
6. Ovid, *Metamorphoses*, Book 3.
7. Sophocles, *Oedipus Rex*, 316.
8. Hippocrates, *The Seed*, 4.
9. Hippocrates, *The Seed*, 4.
10. Hippocrates, *The Seed*, 4.
11. Aristophanes, *Lysistrata*, 130.
12. Aristophanes, *Lysistrata*, 100–150.
13. Aristophanes, *Lysistrata*, 42.
14. Aristophanes, *Lysistrata*, 100–150.
15. Aristophanes, *The Assembly Women*, 465.
16. Haskell Smith, *Rude Talk in Athens*, p. 37.
17. Haskell Smith, *Rude Talk in Athens*, p. 40.
18. Haskell Smith, *Rude Talk in Athens*, p. 41.
19. Plato, *Laws*, XI.
20. Ibid.
21. Ibid.
22. Aristotle, *Politics*, Book XVI.
23. Aristotle, *Politics*, Book XVI.
24. Aristophanes, *Lysistrata*, 119.
25. Aristophanes, *The Assembly Women*.
26. Herodas, *The Scarlet Dildo*, 30.

27. This is Object 202175 on the Beazely Archive Pottery Database, which provides this description.
28. Aristophanes, *Lysistrata*, 217.
29. This particular translation is by Ian Johnston at Vancouver Island University, Nanaimo, BC, Canada.
30. Plato, *Palatine Anthology*, 9.506.
31. Aelian, *Fragment 187/190* (from Stobaeus 3.29.58).
32. Catullus, 5.
33. Catullus, 58.
34. Sappho, fragment 41v.
35. Sappho, 49v.
36. Sappho, 161v.
37. Sappho, 94lp.
38. Sappho, 31v.
39. Plutarch, *Life of Lycurgus*, 18.4.
40. Plutarch, *Sayings of Spartan Women*, Gyrtias 1.
41. *Magical Papyrus*, PGM VII. 423–428.
42. *Magical Papyrus*, PGM VII. 149–154.
43. *Hawara*, P 312 = PGM 32; translation from Brooten, *Love Between Women*, p. 78.
44. *PSI* I 28 = *Suppl.Mag.* I 42; translation Brooten, *Love Between Women*, pp. 84–86.

Chapter 15: Rape and Sexual Assault

1. As defined in the Cambridge Online Dictionary https://dictionary.cambridge.org
2. Hesiod, *Works and Days*, 465–478.
3. Hesiod, *Works and Days*, 293–319.
4. Meander, *The Woman from Samos*.
5. Aristophanes, *The Acharnians*, 334.
6. As per the Cambridge Online Dictionary.
7. Lysias, *On the Murder of Eratosthenes*, 33.
8. Lysias, *On the Murder of Eratosthenes*, 4.
9. Plutarch, *Life of Solon*, 23.
10. Plutarch, *Life of Solon*, 23.
11. Gortyn Code, II.
12. Herodotus, *Histories*, 2.131–2.
13. Pausanias, *Guide to Greece*, 9.13.5.

Chapter 16: Prostitution

1. Sexual Offences Act 2003.
2. Athenaeus, *The Deipnosophists*, 13.569.
3. Xenophon, *Memorabilia*, 2.2.4.
4. Romans like to leave their mark wherever they go by scrawling all over the walls. There are over 100 examples of graffiti scrawled on the walls of one Pompeii brothel that leave no ambiguity as to the function of the building.
5. Strabo, *Geography*, 8.6.20.
6. Bible, *The New Testament*, Acts 9.
7. Bible, *The New Testament*, Corinthians 6.
8. Plutarch, *Life of Solon*, 23.1.

9. Vrisimtzis, *Love, Sex and Marriage in Ancient Greece*, 1019.
10. Plutarch, *Life of Pericles*, 24.2.
11. Plutarch, *Life of Pericles*, 24.1.
12. Plutarch, Life of *Pericles*, 24.2.
13. Plutarch, *Life of Pericles*, 24.3.
14. Plutarch, *Life of Pericles*, 24.6.
15. Plutarch, *Life of Pericles*, 24.6.
16. It's museum object number 1836,0224.173 on the British Museum collection website.
17. This satyr orgy scene is apparently to be found in Berlin Altes Museum.
18. Demosthenes, *Against Neaera*, 59.111.
19. Demosthenes, *Against Neaera*, 59.114.
20. Demosthenes, *Against Neaera*, 59.30.
21. Demosthenes, *Against Neaera*, 59.18.
22. Demosthenes, *Against Neaera*, 59.30.
23. Demosthenes, *Against Neaera*, 59.33.
24. Ibid.
25. Demosthenes, *Against Neaera*, 59.39.
26. Demosthenes, *Against Neaera*, 59.122I.
27. Demosthenes, *Against Neaera*, 59.46.
28. Demosthenes, *Against Neaera*, 59.122.

Part IV: Love Is a Complicated Thing

Chapter 17: And Finally, to Love

1. Pliny the Elder, *The Natural Histories*, ix.152.
2. Pliny the Elder, *The Natural Histories*, xiv70.
3. Pliny the Elder, *The Natural Histories*, vi.54.
4. Pliny the Elder, *The Natural Histories*, xxxvi.20. Cnidas is situated in what is now Turkey.
5. Antipater, *Greek Anthology*, XVI.168.
6. Pliny the Elder, *The Natural Histories*, xxxvi.21.
7. Hesiod, *Theogony*, 176–205.
8. Hesiod, *Theogony*, 213.
9. Homer, *Odyssey*, 4.261.
10. Theognidea, 1386–9.
11. Xenophon, *Symposium*, 8.9.
12. Xenophon, *Symposium*, 8.9.
13. Hesiod, *Theogony*, 119.
14. Fragment 413.
15. James Davidson, *The Greeks and Greek Love*, p. 14.
16. Plato, *Cratylus*, 400d and 419e–420b.
17. Nonnus, *Dionysiaca*, 47. 442 ff.
18. *Magical Papyri*, PGM VII. 405–6.
19. *Magical Papyri*, PGMIV. 1390–1495.
20. *Magical Papyri*, PGM VII. 199–201.
21. *Magical Papyri*, PGM IV. 2708–84.
22. *Magical Papyri*, PGM XXXVI. 333–60.
23. *Magical Papyri*, PGM W. 296–466.

24. *Magical Papyri*, PGM W. 296–466.
25. Demosthenes, *Against Aristogeiton*, 25.79.
26. Plato, *Symposium*, 178.
27. Plato, *Symposium*, 184.
28. Plato, *Symposium*, 193.
29. Plato, *Symposium*, 193.

Bibliography

Aristophanes, *Lysistrata/The Acharnians/The Clouds*, translated by Alan H. Sommerstein (Penguin Classics, 1989)
Aristophanes, *The Assembly Women* (The Internet Classics Archive)
Aristophanes, *The Knights*, translated by Gilbert Murray (George Allen and Unwin, 1956)
Aristotle, *Complete Works* (ATN Publishing, 2025)
Arrian, *The Anabasis of Alexander*, translated by E. J. Chinnock (Hodder and Stoughton, 1884)
Beard, Mary, *Women and Power* (Profile Books, 2017)
Betz, Hans Dieter (ed.), *The Greek Magical Papyri* (University of Chicago Press, 1986)
Bonfante, Larissa, 'The NAKED GREEK', *Archaeology*, vol. 43, no. 5, 1990, pp. 28–35
Carey, C., 'Rape and Adultery in Athenian Law', *The Classical Quarterly*, vol. 45, no. 2, 1995, pp. 407–417
Cartledge, Paul, *Aristophanes and His Theatre of the Absurd* (Bristol Classical Press, 2008)
Cartledge, Paul, *The Spartans* (Macmillan, 2003)
Catullus, *The Shorter Poems*, translated by John Godwin (Oxbow Books, 2007)
Chrystal, Paul, *Women in Ancient Greece* (Fonthill Media Limited, 2017)
Cohen, David, 'Seclusion, Separation, and the Status of Women in Classical Athens', *Greece & Rome*, vol. 36, no. 1, 1989, pp. 3–15
Colden, Mark, *Greek Sport and Social Status* (University of Texas, 2008)
Cole, Myke, *The Bronze Lie* (Osprey Publishing, 2021)
Davidson, James, *The Greeks and Greek Love* (Phoenix, 2007)
Dean-Jones, Lesley, 'Menstrual Bleeding According to the Hippocratics and Aristotle', *Transactions of the American Philological Association (1974–)*, vol. 119, 1989, pp. 177–191
Demosthenes, *Against Neaera*, translated by Norman W. DeWitt (Harvard University Press, 1949)
Dickie, Matthew, *Magic and Magicians in The Graeco-Roman World* (Routledge, 2001)
Dover, K. J., *Greek Homosexuality* (Bloomsbury Academic, 2016)
Euripides, *The Bacchae and Other Plays* (Penguin Classics, 2006)
Forster, E. M., *Maurice* (Adage Book House, 2024)
Galen, *Selected Works*, translated by P. N. Singer (Oxford University Press, 1997)
Goldhill, Simon, *Love, Sex and Tragedy: Why Classics Matters* (John Murray, 2004)
Graf, Fritz, *Magic in the Ancient World* (Harvard, 1997)
Haynes, Natalie, *Pandora's Jar: Women in Greek Myths* (Picador, 2020)
Herondas, *Mimes*, translated by M. S. Buck (1921)
Hippocratic Writings, translated by Professor Geoffrey Earnest Richard Lloyd (Penguin Books, 1983)
Isaeus, *On the Estate of Pyrrhus*, translated by Edward Seymor Forster (Harvard University Press, 1962)
Johnson, Marguerite, *Sexuality in Greek and Roman Society in Literature* (Routledge, 2022)

Kershaw, Stephen (ed.), *The Penguin Dictionary of Classical Mythology* (Penguin Books, 1991)
Keuls, Eva C., *The Reign of the Phallus* (University of California Press, 1985)
Konstan, David, *Beauty, the Fortunes of an Ancient Greek* (Oxford University Press, 2014)
Llewellyn-Jones, Lloyd, 'House and Veil in Ancient Greece', *British School at Athens Studies*, vol. 15, 2007, pp. 251–258
Lysias, *On the Murder of Eratosthenes*, translated by W. R. M. Lamb (Harvard University Press, London, 1930)
Macgillivray, Alexander J., *Minotaur: Sir Arthur Evans and the Archaeology of the Minoan Myth* (Pimlico, 2001)
Meander, *The Arbitration and Samia*
Miller, Stephen G., *Ancient Greek Athletics* (Yale University Press, 2004)
Neer, Richard T, *Art and Archaeology of the Greek World* (Thames and Hudson, 2012)
Pausanias, *Guide to Greece*, translated by Peter Levi (Penguin Classics, 1971)
Philostratus, *Gymnasticus* (Loeb, Harvard University Press, 2014)
Plato, *The Complete Works of Plato*, translated by Benjamin Jowett (ATOZ Classics, 2018)
Pliny the Elder, *Natural History: A Selection*, translated by John Healey (Penguin Books, 1991)
Plutarch, *The Complete Works*, translated by Bernadotte Perrin (Strelbytskyy Multimedia Publishing, 2021)
Poliakoff, Michael B., *Combat Sports in the Ancient World* (Yale University Press, 1987)
Pomeroy, Sarah B., *Goddesses, Whores, Wives and Slaves: Women in Classical Antiquity* (Pimlico, 1994)
Robson, James, *Sex and Sexuality in Classical Athens* (Edinburgh University Press, 2013)
Sappho, *Stung with Love: Poems and Fragments*, translated by Aaron Poochigian (Penguin Books, 2025)
Stehle, Eva, 'The Body and Its Representations in Aristophanes' *Thesmophoriazousai*: Where Does the Costume End?' *The American Journal of Philology*, vol. 123, no. 3, 2002, pp. 369–406
Sophocles, *Antigone/Oedipus the King/Electra*, translated by H. D. F. Kitto (Oxford World Classics, 2008)
Soranus, *Gynaecology* (Baltimore John Hopkins Press, 1956)
Suetonius, *The Twelve Caesars*, translated by Robert Graves (Penguin Classics, 1999)
The Three Trials of Oscar Wilde: www.famous-trials.com/wilde
Thucydides, *History of the Peloponnesian War*, translated by Richard Crawley (Everyman, 1993)
Walcot, P., 'Greek Attitudes towards Women: The Mythological Evidence', *Greece & Rome*, vol. 31, no. 1, 1984, pp. 37–47
Xenophon, *Complete Works*, translated by Carleton L. Brownson (Delphi Ancient Classics, 2013)

Index